Assisting Seniors at Home

ASSISTING SENIORS AT HOME

A Planning Guide
for Families and Caregivers

Gretchen Mary Rose

Occupational Therapist Registered, Licensed

294050

About the Author

A graduate of Wayne State University (Detroit), author Gretchen Mary Rose has years of clinical experience in behavioral medicine and physical disabilities rehabilitation. In her therapeutic work with clients from young adults to seniors she has demonstrated the value of including the arts and music as therapeutic and motivating factors in individualized care planning. Soon after she became an independent health care consultant in 2002, she recognized the need for a team approach — a "care group" — in the service of seniors in their homes. Out of her personal experience and her wider research into current trends in senior care at home she has produced a unique planning guide to serve the needs of families, caregivers, and seniors.

Acknowledgments

The author is grateful to Thomas P. Fenton and Mary J. Heffron for their editorial, design, and production guidance and to Rita Rose Zyber and Patricia A. Robinson for additional editorial assistance.
Illustrations: Gretchen Mary Rose
Cover photograph: Michael Robinson

ISBN-13: 978-1511432207
ISBN-10: 1511432209

Note: This book is not intended as a substitute for professional medical advice. Always consult a medical professional regarding any changes noted in physical and/or behavioral performance exhibited by the client for whom in-home care services may be provided.

Contents

Introduction

MANY OLDER ADULTS ARE CHOOSING TO LIVE AT HOME as long as possible. Today, numerous options and support systems exist allowing seniors the opportunity to enjoy the independence and security of their own homes for longer periods of time. As seniors choose to age at home, they may need a team of support people as health declines. The dynamics of the team-care process and making the senior's home a safe, energy efficient setting for long-term care are outlined in this book. The information presented will be helpful to anyone in the responsible role of caring for an aging person. Topics included are: hiring caregivers, harmonizing responsibilities and establishing a healthy, supportive daily routine within the home. Home modifications for safety and accessibility are highlighted as well. The focus of this book is threefold, *hiring private caregivers* who will serve the *needs of the senior* in *coordination with the family*, with suggestions for role delineations and specific duties that each team member will perform. The Appendix presents templates to copy and formulate care plans from the perspective of a team approach.

In regard to more complex care at home, such as for those seniors who have multiple diagnoses or limitations resulting from cerebral vascular accident, closed head injury, or paraplegic/quadriplegic involvement, further education and training is recommended. Care provision, at home in these circumstances, is not within the scope of information provided in this resource.

The information presented in this book is not intended to be used as a substitute for medical advice. The senior's health care needs and medication regime remain under the direction of the primary care physician. Always consult the senior's medical doctor as physical or behavioral changes occur.

Although family members are recognized as primary caregivers, the term caregiver as used in this book will refer to hired private care providers, not family members, in an effort to define each role separately even though responsibilities overlap.

Chapter 1

The Aging Process

HEALTHY AGING BEGINS WITH A WHOLESOME LIFESTYLE and self-care routine early in life. Yet even with these sound measures in place, the natural progression of aging challenges stability, mentally and physically, and thus requires continual adjustments toward managing decline.

Assistance will become necessary when an elder family member begins to exhibit signs of cognitive losses, decreased physical endurance, or behaviors with marked changes in personality. A cascade of emotional reactions by both the senior and family members occurs. For the senior a loss of independence is poignant. Family members may hold negative feelings regarding the changes exhibited by the senior. Stress compounds as the levels of assistance required by the senior for safety and management of self-care increase. Grief and anger will be part of the natural response. All of these emotions are normal reactions. Geriatric doctors and professional counselors provide guidance. Local programs such as the Area Agency on Aging, local senior centers, and hospitals may be able to assist as the family adapts to the changing needs of the senior.

Cost Concerns

Along with emotional stress comes the question of how to pay for care. Even the best retirement plans may not meet the reality of the cost of healthcare management as one ages. The family will face difficult decisions in the search for the most practical directions to take. Care options may include assisted living centers, skilled nursing facilities, day care providers, or, if the senior remains at home, hired care providers. Hiring an in-home caregiver may help to keep costs manageable, while maintaining a good quality of life for the senior.

Before making major decisions, family members should consider various options.

> Request a visit from home healthcare providers recommended by the primary care physician to determine the senior's functioning level and if the senior will be safe at home. See Chapter 2, "The Caregiving Team," for more information about the role of the home healthcare providers.
> Examine all options available outside of the senior's home: assisted living programs, county services, long-term care facilities, agencies providing caregiving services.
> Visit facility websites or care provider agencies to research and gather information.
> Examine options available for care at home: ask friends, or someone you know in local organizations or church communities, for references regarding private in-home caregivers.
> Determine a practical course within financial means; consult elder care lawyers to assist in planning and management of the cost of long-term care, as well as advanced directives.
> Engage help, attend educational seminars and support groups.

Early Intervention

If the family determines the senior will be able to live safely at home with a caregiver and family support, early intervention is recommended while the senior is active and semi-independent. Early intervention will allow both the senior and family time to become comfortable with a caregiver and a health maintenance routine at home before independence decreases.

Seniors who have assistance at the earliest stages of decline demonstrate a healthy adjustment to aging due to the psychological support gleaned from regular visits provided early on. At these beginning levels of care, when a parent is semi-independent, a caregiver may be needed to help with errands, grocery shopping, heavy housecleaning or companionship visits on a minimal schedule. It is important that early intervention is care-

fully interfaced with the senior's routine. The active, semi-independent senior may resent the intrusion of a caregiver when they feel healthy. It is
imperative that the care team respects the senior's active level of functioning and offer assistance, only, for the tasks the senior cannot manage.

Early intervention also includes the establishment of advanced directives on behalf of the senior's wishes. The process of formulating advanced
directives will be guided by a lawyer with an expertise in elder law. This
representative will help the family and senior establish a twofold process.
One is to determine who will make medical decisions based upon the senior's expressed wishes, called a health care agent or a patient advocate.
Two is to select someone who will manage the senior's financial matters,
called Durable Power of Attorney for Finances.

These important legal matters must be discussed with the senior while
he/she is able to express wishes regarding sensitive matters, such as, end-
of-life decisions and financial planning/estate management.

Finding Home Care Providers

There are two main avenues from which to select an in-home caregiver:
through agencies that provide care at home or direct hiring of individual
private caregivers.

Caregiving agencies provide services organized from a pool of caregivers. Agencies work within a contract or agreement and determine a specific fee for services needed. Hospitals may recommend agencies for
caregiver provision. Research locally to find an agency that suits the family
and the senior's needs.

An individual private caregiver is a contractor who arrives in the home
for a designated schedule and specific duties. Private caregivers are individuals working independently with a contract or agreement (verbal or
written). This person is usually referred by word-of-mouth from neighbors,
people you know, or other dependable sources, such as community organi-
zations or church groups and would not be affiliated with an agency.

Hiring a Caregiver through an Agency

Hiring a caregiver through an agency has positive as well as negative
aspects. Two *postives* are (1) coverage is maintained even if a worker is sick
or needs to take time off, and (2) assistance from an agency may include a
wide range of resources or service options. On the *negative* side, the caregiver receives only a portion of the hourly wage the family pays. This may
create a disincentive for providing quality care. Additionally, a caregiver
from an agency may change schedule frequently or the person providing
care may vary.

Hiring a Private Caregiver

Hiring a private caregiver also has positive and negative aspects. The *positives* include (1) the same caregiver arrives each day as scheduled with no variations in the person providing care, and (2) the money the family pays a private caregiver goes directly to the person who is providing care, increasing incentive for quality care provision. On the *negative* side, the caregiver may have to take sick days with no alternate coverage and the caregiver may not have a broad range of resources to provide the most thorough service.

If seeking a caregiver from either an agency or a private practitioner, it is recommended that the family consult with an attorney regarding liability for anyone working in the senior's home. It is essential to confirm that the potential caregiver(s) have had a criminal background check, and are bonded or insured. An agency providing caregiving services may have liability coverage/policies in place to consider and discuss prior to employment.

If the choice is a private caregiver for senior care at home, liability insurance must be considered. If the caregiver has Worker's Compensation Insurance, he/she would be covered in case of an injury. If not, do not assume that homeowner's insurance will cover injuries incurred by a hired caregiver while working in the senior's home. If the homeowner's insurance policy does not specify additional risk, the policy may not cover the caregiver. Homeowner's insurance companies will have to add a specific rider clause for the private caregiver if this coverage is not in place. Other considerations are theft insurance or bonding. Also check auto insurance coverage in relation to injury incurred by the caregiver when driving on errands or during senior transport. Accident insurance for other drivers will need to be explored if the caregiver is using the senior's car or a car the family owns.

It is firmly recommended that the family contact the local police department for information regarding a criminal or drug related background check as this is advisable before hiring any care provider, either private or from an agency if the agency does not provide this information.

It is critical to hire dependable, honest caregivers who will carry out the required designated responsibilities. Impeccable references and careful scrutiny during the interview process will be necessary. Families should ask for a résumé indicating educational level, experience, and any credentials relative to the position.

Interviewing a Private Caregiver

Working with a senior is a private matter. The provision of caregiving services requires skills that demonstrate competence and engender trust. The hired caregiver who is successful will have the ability to form an empathic relationship. Empathy, in regard to the senior, is the ability to understand one who is losing independence, is in pain, or grieving personal and cognitive losses. A caregiver who is able to remain calm and think clearly, through the process of personality changes and declining health, will be a match for this type of work. Successful interpersonal characteristics of a private caregiver are listed below.

Character References of a Supportive Caregiver

› Demonstrate patience, endure challenges without complaint.
› Remain calm when the senior is upset or angry.
› Demonstrate professional behavior. Arriving for work on time is important as the schedules of others on the caregiving team may dovetail.
› Work diplomatically, clearly communicate observations and situations that arise without blame or judgment.
› Work without supervision but not assuming the decision-making level of a family member.
› The caregiver is self-directed in managing his or her duties as specified.
› Are honest and accountable for their actions at all times: provide receipts after shopping for the senior, manage time productively, and adhere to a schedule.
› Understand confidentiality, safeguard the privacy of the senior and family. This means no gossip and no discussion with others of any information regarding the senior or the family.
› Are flexible. This is essential as one works in the uncontrolled environment of the senior's home.
› Are effective communicators, express clearly, that which is observed regarding the senior's ability to manage activities of daily living or any health concerns.
› Are attentive, give the senior full attention while interacting. In general, listen more than talk.
› Are empathic, able to understand a situation from the senior's perspective and become aware of the senior's personal and cultural experience.
› Are good companions, introduce activities and entertainment options that engage the senior, are sensitive to what the senior likes and wants to do.
› Have a sense of business needs and organization. Self-employed caregivers must be able to manage business require-

ments such as income records for taxes, mileage records, and invoicing with accuracy, verifying billable time.

The list above describes attributes one will demonstrate in the caregiving process. The family may use this list to formulate scenarios and questions as they interview prospective candidates. Families should prepare for the interview with questions regarding the senior's specific needs and how the caregiver will intervene. The caregiver's answers should reflect the qualities listed above. This will assist the family and the senior to determine the best care provider. Include the senior as much as possible in the interview process.

Caregiver Service Options

The caregiver's training credentials and qualifications will determine the job description he/she will fill. The following list identifies some service options a caregiver may offer.

> Housekeeping/laundry
> Errands, grocery shopping
> Meal provision; medication reminders/monitoring
> Cooking (food handlers card from county health department is recommended)
> Dressing assistance
> Companionship and cognitive activities (art, games, reading, puzzles, mail interaction)
> Active range-of-motion exercises (guidance from home healthcare providers and doctor's approval)
> Transporting the senior to events (chauffeur's license is recommended)
> Personal ADL's and bathing assistance if résumé indicates adequate training/experience or certified nursing assistant or licensed practical nurse credentials.

Once the caregiver is hired, the senior and family members become *clients* from the caregiver's perspective. Confidentiality, from that moment on, will be maintained to safeguard the privacy of all those involved. Chapter 10, "Professional Performance," has more information regarding confidentiality and the caregiver's character references.

The information provided above gives a general outline of the issues that need to be considered as the family seeks out and hires in-home caregivers. Legal constraints and insurance procedures vary from state to state, as well as regulations formulated to guide agencies providing caregiving services. Seek out exact guidelines for the local area in which the caregiving services will be provided.

The aging continuum presents challenges for the family and the senior. For many families, the first choice in managing the aging process is care at home. The information presented in this book will help determine if care at home is the most practical course to take as parents age. The following chapters outline information and suggestions to help solve problems encountered on this journey, including senior skill levels as observed in the decline process.

Chapter 2

The Caregiving Team

THE SUPPORT TEAM AT HOME consists of the senior, primary care physician, family and hired caregivers. The roles of each member of the team will need to be identified with specific duties assigned. The credentials that the caregiver brings to the support team will determine the level of care he/she will provide. Expectations of the private caregiver beyond his/her scope of training would be contraindicated. Role delineations for those involved in the caregiving process will eliminate misunderstandings and decrease stress. Responsibilities may change, but commitment, mutual support, and reliability are qualities expected from both family members and hired caregivers for a successful outcome.

Experts recommend hiring a caregiver early on if possible. This allows both senior and family enough time to become comfortable with a new person before independence decreases. Early intervention also includes an evaluation of the senior's level of functioning and home safety requirements. The senior's primary care physician or geriatric specialist can prescribe home healthcare providers for this preliminary evaluation.

Home healthcare providers are a group of professionals usually consisting of a registered nurse, social worker, occupational and physical therapists, and in some cases, a speech-language pathologist. The home healthcare providers will give the senior and family valuable information regarding the senior's level of function in areas of self-care: grooming/hygiene, dressing, meal preparation, referred to as activities of daily living (ADL's); and structural adjustments (home modifications) for environmental safety. They will recommend equipment such as grab bars in the bathroom and bedroom, support measures in the kitchen, as well as adaptive equipment the senior will need to live as independently as possible. A registered nurse will manage the medication process (including how and when to dispense medications) and will answer questions regarding side effects. A social worker will connect the family with community support systems and will assist with emotional adjustments as changes occur. The role of the home healthcare providers is limited; visits last about two to three weeks, one to two times a week.

Team Participants

For the senior who remains at home, the caregiving team is as follows
   › The primary care physician or geriatric specialist directs the medical process, provides medication and referrals as needed, such as, home healthcare providers, or specialists.
   › The home healthcare providers determine the senior's level of function in activities of daily living and recommend safety requirements for the home environment.
   › The senior and family are the directors of the care process at home. Family members formulate the day-to-day Care Plan with the senior.
   › Family members maintain the home as a safe, clean living space.
   › A primary contact person, ideally a family member, manages communications with the team.
   › Hired caregivers will provide support and manage day-to-day duties as specified in the Care Plan per qualifications, as well as maintain a safe, clean living space.
The family and hired caregiver(s) will be closely involved with the senior on a daily basis. A successful team will work coordinately to provide visitation coverage for the senior and services as required.

How the Team Works

Each team member has specific responsibilities. Family members will organize the home milieu for safety, based upon the primary care physician's recommendations and information from the home healthcare providers. The senior will have responsibilities to manage within his/her functional skill level and safety parameters as determined by the home healthcare pro-viders. The primary contact person and the hired caregiver will structure a schedule with specific visiting hours and responsibilities directly related to the senior's needs. The family and the hired caregiver will identify services he/she is qualified to provide and the hours available. From this coordi-nated effort, a Care Plan is formulated. Ideally this team will support each other in the caregiving process with the broad goal identified as senior care at home.

Family members at a distance are an important part of the team as well. A son or daughter may be able to manage the parent's financial matters and pay bills automatically from a long-distance location. Grandchildren, nie-ces, and nephews can write cards or letters. Family members who visit from afar may want to stagger visits to provide much needed respite time for sib-lings who provide day-to-day caregiving. Vacations may be planned where the out-of-state siblings become temporary caregivers to help offset the stress for those who live close.

Establishing a Care Plan

Successful assistance for the senior at home requires an organized ap-proach for smooth and consistent care. Once the caregiver is hired, and the senior's skill level is identified, the team can sit down and create a Care Plan.

The Care Plan spells out who will do what in the process of caring for the senior. This will assure that all aspects of need are identified and as-signed to someone on the team (family, senior or hired caregiver). The visit-ing schedule will also be established.

In the following chapter three tools are outlined to assist the family in structuring and applying a Care Plan based on the senior's needs.

The *Team Care Planning Guide* works as a blueprint to identify the du-ties of the family members, contact person(s), the hired caregiver(s) and the senior.

The *Skill Level Indicator* marks specific signs of decline in the senior's skill level.

The *Care Plan* is derived from the above tools. This is the job descrip-tion defining the day-to-day assistance provided by the team to serve the needs of the senior.

Chapter 3

Organizing and Adapting a Care Plan

THE INFORMATION IN THIS CHAPTER will introduce three tools: The first two tools are the Team Care Planning Guide and the Skill Level Indicator. These will help to identify responsibilities and formulate job descriptions for each person on the team. The third tool, the Care Plan, is found in the Appendix. Make a copy of the Care Plan and record the services your senior family member will need as determined from the first two tools. This book suggests family members as the key role players. However, significant others or friends of the family may be assigned as responsible partners in the team organization, especially in the situation where all family members live at a distance. Team leaders will be identified as a primary and secondary contact person, as well as someone assigned to manage doctors' appointments and medication, possibly the health care advocate. The senior will manage tasks within his/her skill level. Revisit the Skill Level Indicator as the senior's skill's decline to restructure the Care Plan relative to the changing needs.

The Team Care Planning Guide

Family members are ultimately responsible for the care and safe environment of the senior. If possible, regular conferences for the team are recommended. The directors of the team will be family members, as well as the senior. Team member assignments are detailed below.

Contact Person

A primary contact person will be determined as the team leader. A secondary contact person will need to be assigned if the primary is unavailable. The contact person, family and senior will specify the services required from the hired caregiver and formulate an agreement and a designated schedule.

> Contact person will be the hired caregiver's guide throughout the care process.
> The contact person will intervene with emergencies as required.
> Contact person or family member is responsible for providing alternate coverage in the event that the caregiver is absent.
> Family member or contact person arranges conferences to problem solve and make changes in the Care Plan as needed.

Communications

The team will identify and use specific communications tools. It is recommended that some form of daily documentation be provided by the caregiver. See the Appendix for an example of a documentation check list.

A large communications calendar should be placed where each team member can see the month in advance. This will list appointments for the senior, the caregiver's schedule, as well as times the primary contact person may be out of town. Emergency phone numbers, the phone number of a trusted repair person, and e-mail addresses may be attached at the calendar as well as placed by the phone.

The contact person is the hub of communications. It is helpful to set up a form of group networking in regard to dispatching information as the senior's needs change. Health or home concerns may happen quickly and a dependable message system will assure a response. Some suggestions are group e-mails, or devise a process where siblings call the next family member and share information dispatched by the contact person. In addition, the contact person has the following assignments.

> Contact person is responsible for communicating any changes in schedule for senior care with other family members and caregiver.
> If the primary contact person is unavailable, the secondary contact person will be assigned as guide for problem solving or emergency situations.
> Contact person will set up a medical alert system for the senior

who lives alone and give instructions to the senior and the team regarding how to use it.

› Contact person will alert the caregiver and team of any safety precautions regarding the senior's health history or changes in health status per doctor's recommendations.

Health Care Advocate

It is recommended that doctor appointments and handling medications are assigned to a family member, or the health care advocate if the senior is unable to do this independently. Direct communications with the senior's doctor by a family member or advocate is the best means by which to manage the senior's health care and medication.

› A designated family member or health care advocate will make doctor appointments for the senior and meet all doctors involved.

› The health care advocate will communicate the specific date/time of appointments, mark them on the communications calendar, and adjust the caregiver's schedule as needed.

› The advocate will let the primary physician know about medications prescribed by other doctors or specialists involved in the senior's care.

› A current medication list as well as specific food or medication allergies will be provided to the team by the one assigned to manage medications for emergency purposes.

› The advocate will alert the team of any changes in the senior's health, medications, or safety precautions required per a doctor's recommendations.

› A designated family member or health care advocate is responsible for the management of medication refills.

The family will determine how the medication will be administered. It is recommended that a family member prepare the medication pack per doctor's orders and provide specific instructions for others on the team to follow/administer. In some circumstances, the local Area Agency on Aging may provide the services of a registered nurse who will visit to assist the family in the safe dispensing of medications. This will enhance the understanding of side effects and issues involved in drug interactions.

Household Maintenance

Household maintenance is a family responsibility. All team members will communicate any problems observed in the climate, household building structure, and general environment, and assist in maintaining a clean,

safe living space.
> Family will set up the senior's home for safe long-term care. See Chapter 6, "Accessibility and Safety in the Home."
> Family is responsible for seasonal climate control and security systems.
> Family will respond to any reported home maintenance repairs that are needed.
> Family is responsible to keep entrance/exit open (snow removal) for emergency rescue team or for the senior's escape plan in case of a house fire.
> Family is responsible for establishing a fire escape plan and to assist the senior in practicing this plan once a week. Caregiver will take part in this practice.
> Family will place smoke and carbon monoxide detectors in the home and provide safety checks frequently to be sure they are operating correctly.
> Family is responsible for including a rider on homeowner's insurance policy to cover any injury incurred by the caregiver in the senior's home, as well as valuable items.
> Family will remove valuables or secure them in a locked compartment, if moveable.

Caregiver Assignments

The hired caregiver will have specific duties/assignments based on skill level and training. The caregiver is a team member who will provide support services as identified at the first interview with the family. This person may serve all of the needs of the senior from housekeeping to personal grooming/hygiene as qualified.
> Caregiver will identify services he/she is qualified to provide.
> Caregiver, family and senior will identify and assign specific duties for the caregiver and set up a visiting schedule.
> Caregiver will be responsible for his/her scheduled hours and duties as determined.
> Caregiver will complete documentation as the team requires.
> Caregiver will establish a helpful supportive working relationship with the senior and family.
> Caregiver will alert the contact person of any home maintenance repairs needed.
> Caregiver will alert the contact person of any problems or injuries exhibited by the senior.
> Caregiver will get information from the family regarding how

to manage emergencies.

> Family will provide a list of the senior's allergies, and medications.

> Family will provide specific emergency instructions if a "Do Not Resuscitate Order" is in place, per senior's wishes; or if hospice is part of the care-provision team.

> Caregiver will call 911 or initiate specific emergency intervention in case of injuries or life threatening situations. Caregiver will call contact person following the 911 call.

> Caregiver may remind the senior to take medications as directed by the one designated to monitor medication, following doctor's orders.

> Caregiver will document the medication the senior takes, the time at which it was taken, and assurance that the senior actually took it.

> Caregiver will document any changes in the medication process, such as, if the senior is not willing to take medication. Caregiver will alert the contact person if this occurs.

> The caregiver will alert the one who manages the medication if a refill is needed before medication runs out.

Visiting Schedule

Private caregivers depend on a steady schedule for a stable, reliable income. Situations in the family or senior's life may create long lengths of time when the senior is out of the local area. The family may set up seasonal trips in which the senior is visiting someone out of state for weeks at a time. If a hospitalization should become necessary, the senior may be admitted in-patent or on a rehabilitation unit for many weeks. In that event, proactive plans must be discussed regarding the caregiver's schedule. The caregiver will determine how long he/she is able to leave scheduled time open while waiting for the senior to return home. If budget allows the family may want to provide a retainer fee to support the caregiver during this non-service provision time. This will assure continuity of care and that the caregiver remains part of the team when the senior returns home.

In some cases, the family or the senior may cancel caregiver's hours frequently without justification. If this occurs, the caregiver will need to consider discontinuation of services to maintain financial security. Reasonable cancellations would be for doctor appointments managed by a family memer. Other cancellations may occur for special family gatherings. These may not be frequent.

In summary, the Team Care Planning Guide, as outlined above, is a preliminary reference that may be used to prepare the Care Plan. The Team Care Planning Guide provides a rough draft of job descriptions and identifies duties that need to be addressed in relation to senior care. It suggests possible candidates who may fulfill these responsibilities and prepares the home for a safe caregiving process.

Families will find the best team members suited to carry out the assignments. The senior will direct the Care Plan as much as possible while good health prevails. In some cases, helpers may not be family members but friends or other significant people who may become part of the caregiving team.

Skill Level Indicator

Change is inevitable in the aging population. The second tool outlined in this chapter is the Skill Level Indicator. This tool will help the team identify the senior's functional level as changes occur.

The skills of the senior will not be determined by the team alone. The primary care physician or geriatric doctor will verify and provide guidance through the visiting home healthcare providers. Assessments from these professionals will help the family set up safety boundaries as required, as well as the amount of assistance the senior will need to complete essential daily activities.

Healthcare practitioners assess one's ability to manage personal health, household needs, engage in social activities, shop within a budget and uphold financial responsibilities. These activities, require the capability to plan, organize and manage time. As health declines, the aging person will show signs of losing these higher functional skills, yet will continue to operate, marginally, in the areas of self-care, such as bathing, grooming and hygiene, dressing, eating, (basic ADL's).

When a senior's planning and organizing skills wane, it is a turning point at which he/she will need assistance. This presents evidence that early intervention is favorable. A caregiver hired early on will bridge the gap between higher level skills: time management, planning, organizing, and basic ADL's.

The Skill Level Indicator is a general guideline to mark various functional stages observed in the aging population. This tool will help the family and primary care physician identify behaviors that mark decline. The Skill Level Indicator will have significant value in adapting the Care Plan proactively as changes occur. It can also be used to determine improvements in the senior's functional level.

The Skill Level Indicator outlines four distinct levels of functioning that the senior will exhibit in the decline process. This guide notes specific behaviors that mark skill loss as the senior demonstrates changes in aptitude or stamina.

Level 1

The senior family member is living at home independently with a spouse, significant other or alone. She/he enjoys social engagements outside of the home with a lifestyle rich in quality. Mental and physical health are stable with the support of regular exercise, a good diet and/or medication.

› Senior is able to walk to and from car and drives for errands and social engagements.
› Senior is functioning in all levels of personal self-care, nutrition and basic housekeeping; may need domestic help for heavy housecleaning and/or yard work.
› Senior manages finances and is able to shop for necessities within budget.
› Senior plans and attends activities, sets appointments with the doctor.
› Takes medication as prescribed independently and engages in exercise/health routine.

A person at this level is living the golden years of retirement with good health mentally and physically and enough stamina to engage in life as much as possible.

Level 2

One at this level will present with the beginning stages of health decline, possibly both mentally and physically. For one who lives alone, this is a time when most accidents may happen due to unexpected loss of skill or stamina. Introducing precautionary measures, such as a medical alert system and regular visits/frequent phone calls, will bring peace of mind for the senior and family. Social support is vital to maintain health. Seniors at this level may need assistance for tasks that require planning, organizing and time management as these skills begin to decline.

› Senior is able to ambulate in the home with a cane or walker, needs a clutter free environment and open floor space to prevent falls.
› Senior may be able to use home appliances such as laundry washer/dryer for light loads if the appliances are located on the main floor.
› Senior is able to access most items needed to prepare meals and is able to use stove, oven, or microwave safely.

> Senior demonstrates decrease in stamina for most tasks. Continence begins to fail.
> Senior may have intermittent lapses in time management to sustain proper nutrition, medications, grooming/hygiene needs and responsibility for events or appointments.
> Senior may need encouragement or assistance from others to engage in social events outside the home.
> Senior needs a hired housekeeper to manage deep cleaning, plus help with grocery shopping, lifting items.
> Senior may need help to set up doctor appointments; may still drive but only as weather permits.

Frequent visits from family or friends will provide support and decrease isolation. Close monitoring will assure that the senior is safe. The family may begin to install home modifications for safe accessibility, toilet transfers and walking. The home healthcare providers will advise on the need for grab bars in bathroom/bedroom. Railings on both sides of the stairs will assist one in reaching the upper level safely. If the senior's bedroom/bathroom is on an upper level, a separate cane at the top of the stairs will be helpful (or a walker if used). If possible, consider moving bed and bathroom to one-level living accommodations. An emergency medical alert system must be put in place if not set up previously.

Kitchen will be set up with meal preparation items in reachable cupboards with easy accessibility to assure successful task completion. Small cooking pots for one or two people can replace large food preparation items/utensils. A kitchen stool at the counter, or a chair at the table for preparing meals will promote energy conservation. Adaptive equipment, such as a reacher, special cutting/chopping tools in the kitchen, may help maintain independence if the senior is able to follow instructions to use these tools safely. Monitoring will be needed around nutrition needs, use of stove/oven and correct medication protocol. Any difficulty noted in nutrition, use of appliances and medication management by the senior is an indication of decline and may require increased assistance in these areas.

Laundry room will also need accessibility adaptations for energy conservation. A counter or table will serve as a folding platform. Small loads may be within the senior's skill level, yet assistance may be needed in moving items to/from laundry room. Use small containers to hold laundry detergent for easy use.

Interviewing for a caregiver at this time is recommended to promote early intervention while the senior is able to learn and practice safety habits and adjust to a new person in his/her support group.

Monitor and discuss driving safety with the primary care physician at this stage.

Level 3

Time management, planning and organizing skills begin to fail. More support from the caregiving team will become necessary if care at home continues. The focus for the senior is on managing basic activities of daily living.

> Senior is ambulating with walker, or may need a wheelchair.
> Physical strength is diminished as noted in lack of ability to complete some self-care tasks such as laundry, bathing, grooming/hygiene, nutritional meal preparation and medication regime.
> Ability to rise from a chair or toilet is labored and difficult.
> Upper limb, hand strength and dexterity are noted as decreased in that the senior exhibits difficulty lifting items from cupboards such as pots/pans or canned goods.
> Opening jars or heavily wrapped food items are almost impossible.
> Thoughts expressed may be off topic and repeated, memory deficits are noted.
> The senior may become lost if he/she leaves home unescorted.
> Evidence of cognitive decline may be noted in how items in the house lack organization, for example, dishes in cupboards may be dirty. Important events may be forgotten.

A senior at this level should not live alone. One-level living arrangements and home modifications such as grab bars in the bathroom, at the bedside, and at stairways or entrances will provide safe living accommodations. Any unused stairways should be blocked off and locked. A ramp from the entrance to the car will be needed if one is in a wheelchair.

The caregiver will provide assistance as needed, in some, or all steps of bathing, dressing, grooming/hygiene. Specific education and training is recommended for the caregiver as the senior's health declines and intervention becomes more complex.

Stove top cooking may be limited to the use of a microwave to prevent fire hazard or accidental burns. The senior may join in the process of easy meal preparations with supervision, such as, warm foods or previously prepared meals in microwave, make toast/cereal, add pre-cut fruit to yogurt or cottage cheese. It is helpful to have sandwich items prepared and available like tuna, egg salad, or ham, ready to use with pre-cut cheese. Be sure refrigerated containers are light enough for the senior to handle, such as milk containers, or storage/warming dishes. Electric can openers will allow access to canned goods like soups, vegetables, beans. The pull-top can openers are difficult for some seniors to use.

Escorting a senior out of the house will require training in safe ambulation for one using a walker or wheelchair in the outside environment. This includes how to safely get in and out of the car.

Allow the senior to do as much as possible according to skill level. Safety limitations are a priority. The senior's full energy will be focused on managing basic activities of daily living. Time management and pacing tasks to allow rest periods will be important interventions.

Level 4

Final stages and hospice care follow as the senior's capacity to manage all self-care tasks declines. Twenty-four-hour care at home or in a skilled nursing facility is needed.

At this stage the senior may require
› Oxygen
› Assistance to eat/drink liquids
› Full assistance with incontinence and bowel movement process
› Skin management (turn the senior every 1.5 hours to prevent pressure sores)
› Full assistance in bathing

Special training is required to assist at this stage of care. Two people may be required to assist the senior with bathing. Lift equipment, a medical bed and a wheelchair may be purchased or brought in from a hospice organization, if not incorporated into the routine at a previous level. As vital organs begin to fail, at the final days of the senior's life, the family needs room to be near their dying family member. The hired caregiver will be able to assist in cleanup and support the hospice team. The family and caregivers should engage in counseling after the senior's death. Private journaling during the caregiving process and as one dies is helpful to release emotions.

The skill levels listed in the tool above can help to identify the signs that show a need for change. These skill levels do not include everything that a senior will exhibit. Each individual will go through the aging process in their own manner. Some will move through the levels quickly, others more slowly. Some may not progress to Level 4 and will pass at earlier stages of decline. See more levels of function, specific to those diagnosed with Alzheimer's disease or dementia listed in Chapter 11, "Information regarding Diagnoses."

The tools introduced above—the Team Care Planning Guide, the Skill Level Indicator, and the Care Plan (see Appendix)—will assist the family in formulating a structured, individual service intervention for the senior who lives at home. See Chapter 6, "Accessibility and Safety in the Home," for additional care planning recommendations.

Chapter 4

Applying the Care Plan

THE CARE PLAN will highlight the senior's skill level and indicate the tasks he/she will be able to perform on a daily basis. The Care Plan is applied with respect for the routine the senior has in place. Caregivers offer services, as needed, in coordination with the senior's regular daily activities.

Observing the senior performing tasks in a daily routine will reveal changes in functional level. Caregivers as objective observers, will note behaviors that announce the need for change in the level of care provided. When the senior demonstrates difficulty with tasks that were once easy, it is a clear indicator that change is occurring. If this change is consistent, assistance and safety precautions will be needed relative to the skill that is diminished.

In contrast, seniors may show improvement and adaptations will be needed for a higher level of skill performance. Examples of improvements are:

One gains functional skills as a result of day-to-day support the team provides.

One gains skills as he/she recovers from surgery, or an illness goes into remission.

A Routine Supports Independent Living Skills

A senior who maintains a daily routine will retain confidence in skill aptitude and self-satisfaction through a productive lifestyle. A daily routine
will serve the senior's mental and physical well-being as it provides structure and supports engagement in functional activities. A routine will assist
the senior in self-management of ADL's such as eating nutritious foods, taking medications as prescribed, bathing, grooming and hygiene, exercise
and restful sleep. The senior who works through his/her self-care activities
maintains strength, range-of-motion, flexibility, physical stamina and cognitive clarity. The repetitive nature of managing self-care tasks daily, at
aproxmately the same time, activates memory and supports circadian
rhythms. This also promotes psychological support derived from security,
safety and predictability woven into the senior's lifestyle. If there is no routine or safe responsibilities expected of the senior, there will be no measur-
ing mechanism by which to observe the subtle changes indicating either
loss of skill or improved capabilities. Apathy, a lack of purpose, feeling a
sense of failure or vulnerability will result from diminishing the senior's
role in self-care and daily activities.

The home healthcare providers, and the primary care physician will
give recommendations regarding if it is safe for the senior to live alone with
assistance, or will require 24-hour care. From these recommendations, a
day-to-day routine will evolve using the Care Plan as a guide.

A Structured Yet Flexible Routine

The following diagram presents suggestions in time management
throughout the day in which the senior's tasks will interface with duties
performed by the attending caregiver. This formula reflects the probable activities of one functioning at levels 2 and 3 on the Skill Level Indicator. The
client/caregiver relationship will evolve through the day-to-day routine.
Specific, individual needs will create variations, and days will be structured
more or less based upon the stress levels or medical condition of the senior.

Morning. Caregiver will monitor/assist as needed.

Senior will manage: bathing, grooming/hygiene tasks, breakfast
preparation/eating, as well as medication and oral care. Senior will
engage in walking activity or range-of-motion exercises, as instructed by the ome healthcare providers. Tasks that require stamina should happen in the routine when the client is most energetic.
Include rest periods. Monitor and report labored breathing. Use
blood pressure monitor to note this vital sign. Bathing may not happen every day. Monitor for dry skin.

Midmorning. Caregiver will go shopping for healthy food approximately one time a week to maintain supplies for daily proper nutrition and basic household items. This trip is planned when another person is in the home, if the senior cannot be alone. Caregiver will manage housekeeping tasks daily; deep cleaning once every two weeks, or more often if needed. Begin meal preparations for lunch and dinner. Include plenty of water in the senior's diet. Document the senior's task management and mood. Support self-care task management with complimentary feedback.

Midday. Caregiver will monitor/assist as needed.

Senior will manage: lunch preparation/eating. After lunch both senior and caregiver will begin laundry; engage a cognitive activity or social visiting by phone or internet. A healthy routine might include creative activities, meditation, music, tea time, stretch exercises with a walk. Balance functional activities with relaxation events.

Late afternoon. Caregiver will continue to complete tasks such as housekeeping, laundry or dinner preparation. The senior may need to nap or rest at this time. Caregiver will check to be sure all items the senior needs are accessible, and that the household is maintained within the senior's "mental map." Put vacuum cleaners/cleaning supplies away; furniture is in the same familiar places for safe ambulation.

Evening. Caregiver will monitor/assist as needed.

Senior will manage: dinner preparation/eating and kitchen clean up. Preparation for bed begins with oral care, grooming/hygiene, quiet time before bed to enhance sleep, possibly light reading/soft music. Dim lights.

One day each month family or caregiver may be assigned to organizing drawers, storage cabinets, closets, clean oven/stove, fridge, shop for home maintenane requirements, including tools, office supplies, postage stamps, seasonal items, batteries. Check smoke and carbon monoxide detectors.

Each senior will have individual medical instructions to address on a day-to-day basis, such as diabetes management, taking medication as prescribed, or a personal exercise regime. These will need to be included in the routine and supported as required.

Sleep Habits

Sleep is an important aspect of a healthy routine. The senior whose day is not structured may find sleep patterns are disturbed. As stated above, one must incorporate a coordination of rest periods with activities throughout the day. This type of time management is often not within the senior's functional skills especially at level 3 of the Skill Level Indicator. Daily activity in balance with enough rest, proper nutrition and toilet breaks will promote sleep at night.

A structured routine supports the *activity versus sleep cycle*. This natural biological cycle is monitored automatically by circadian rhythms. Circadian rhythms work automatically based upon an inner clock stimulated by the light and dark variations of day and night. The changing daylight initiates arousal in the morning and sleep at night. Circadian rhythms also promote a need to have specific rest periods set into an active daily routine. A drop in energy at times during the day is to be expected. This dip in circadian rhythms frequently occurs in the afternoon. Within the routine of the senior a nap at a specific time each day should be part of the plan. Naps should be limited to one time a day and last no longer than 30 minutes. Nap time may be longer if one is recovering from illness or rebuilding after surgery. For some a nap during the day may cause poor sleep at night and should be monitored closely.

Engagement in activities of interest in balance with intermittent rest periods will support a good night's sleep. A structured daily routine will pace activities to prevent exhaustion or eliminate sedentary restlessness.

Habits that may cause interrupted sleep include
> A senior's daily routine may have too many sedentary hours spent sitting in a chair.
> A senior taking long naps through the day can expect a restless night.
> Too much stimulating activity through the day and late into the evening will leave some seniors anxious and unable to sleep.
> A lack of social engagement, or isolation may affect sleep quality.
> A senior who sleeps with a light or TV on at night will not reach deep levels of sleep.
> A lack of proper nutrition or dehydration may cause a restless night.

Sleeping with the light or TV on all night is a sign that the senior who lives alone is uncomfortable or non-confident about his/her safety. Safety lights are necessary at night but the room where one sleeps should have only subdued light. Another safety accommodation is an easy turn on switch to use the main light while rising for toilet use at night. Relaxing music that turns off automatically may soothe the senior.

Hunger in the night or a lack of satiation through the day will create anxiety and sleep disturbances. Balanced meals with fruits, vegetables, grains (complex carbohydrates), protein, calcium, water and a vitamin supplement will provide proper nutrition and allow psychological comfort and a restful night's sleep. It is recommended that the senior drink plenty of water early in the day. Fresh drinking water placed on the senior's bedside table will quench thirst through the night. See Food as Fuel in Chapter 11, "Information regarding Diagnoses."

Seniors who live alone often report insomnia. Studies on the topic of isolation, as experienced by older adults living alone, show that there may be a connection between loneliness, poor sleep, increased cardiovascular disease and depression. Also noted is that a lack of sleep may contribute to a loss of energy resulting in an inability to engage in social activities. Then a vicious cycle results as isolation causes sleep disturbances. These health problems may be minimized if social engagement is incorporated as part of the routine for successful elder support.

Identify the senior's interests and favorite social activities. Include the senior as much as possible in family and social outings or visits. Organize engagement in these relaxing events on a regular basis. This will decrease feelings of isolation, assure improved sleep, decrease the probability of an accident, as well as sustain well-being, physically and mentally. This is especially critical as the senior wanes between Skill Level Indicators 2 and 3.

Issues of poor sleep need to be taken seriously due to the risk of accidents for one who is not well rested. Sleeplessness may indicate a need for 24-hour care. Discuss this with the senior's doctor.

Accident Prevention

At times a senior living alone may attempt activities that are too difficult and possibly sustain a fall. Limiting isolation assures that someone is available on a regular basis to prevent accidents. Visitors dropping by on a routine basis can assist with any needs that may arise. Make a habit of asking if anything is needed before leaving the senior's home.

It is through the skill of observation that the caregiver and family members become familiar with the limitations of the senior. Any changes noted in the senior's ability to manage ADL's, as well as problems in the living quarters that may impede walking or accessibility must be reported and corrected. Some struggling is necessary as the senior will find many tasks challenging. However, when the senior is observed to be moving out of the safe base of gravity, as illustrated in Chapter 8, "Body Mechanics and Posture Alignment," will indicate a possible loss of balance and intervention will be required.

As a caregiver or family member prepares to leave the home of a semi-independent senior living alone, it is vital to make safety inspections to assure the environment is free of hazards. The following list refers to those who live at home alone and show skill levels to be in the range of level

2 to level 3 on the Skill Level Indicator. Individual circumstances will require specific check points identified relative to the senior's personal needs
and residential floor plan. *It is vital to put these check points into the caregiving
routine.* Frequent visits and careful assessment will need to be made regularly at this stage (between levels 2 and 3) to be sure the senior is safe at
home alone. This can be a vulnerable time for the elderly. Refer to Chapter
7, " Balance and Ambulation," for additional safeguards to prevent falls.

Safety Checklist

> Be sure all doors and windows are locked and secure.
> Be sure that the senior can unlock and safely exit doors.
> Go over safety steps, use of medical alert system, emergency es-
cape route, emergency or contact phone numbers.
> Be sure the phone is working properly, as well as the medical
alert system.
> Be sure entrance and exit passages, as well as all walkways
around the house are clear for safe ambulation.
> Be sure that nutritional foods are accessible and water is placed
on side table where the senior sits and on the bedside table.
> Be sure that toiletries, warm blankets and night clothes are all
accessible.
> Be sure that all appliances are off and the thermostat is at a cor-
rect level for the season.
> Be sure all cleaning supplies/appliances are in storage to pre-
vent trip hazard.
> Be sure oxygen is working properly and is placed correctly on
the senior (if required).
> Be sure that all lighting is working and emergency backup elec-
tric is in functioning order.

In summary, the caregiving process, as identified through the individual Care Plan, is accomplished through the routine. The daily procedures
listed above are suggested for a successful in-home, team-care approach.
Caregivers, family members, and senior will be responsible for specific duties regarding daily task completion. Assistance will be provided to the senior only as needed. Monitoring safety measures must become part of the
daily routine. A good caregiver will continuously direct the safe practices of
the senior performing ADL's, and be sure all safety check points are secured
when leaving the client's residence.

Chapter 5

Engaging in the Self-Care Process

CAREGIVERS WILL NEED TO MOTIVATE THE SENIOR to complete his/her responsibilities in the daily routine. Techniques to engage the senior may have to be invented based upon the personality of the senior we serve and his/her interests. Family support is an important part of the caregiving process. Encouragement from a spouse, son, daughter or other relatives is invaluable in helping the senior remain motivated to complete his/her self-care duties. For the senior motivation is inspired through the following.

> The need to be safe
> The need to be as independent as possible within skill level parameters
> The desire for quality of life fulfilled by engaging in activities of interest
> Daily management of self-care activities with evidence of accomplishment

Focus on the senior's interests. The senior may show greater motivation if we explain why routine tasks are good for them. Describe how exercises will help them to dress and prepare for a social engagement or other activities they like to do. This will help the senior identify personally with his/her responsibilities and sustain a purposeful lifestyle. Work at the senior's pace within a balance of rest-versus-activity, especially seniors with diseases such as arthritis or fibromyalgia.

Timing is important to gain a positive response from the senior. Present activities with careful planning. Difficult tasks will be more successful if done during the most active part of the senior's day. Assign only a few days a week as the designated times to engage in more difficult routine activities such as showering, washing hair or taking trips out of the house. Remove distractions. Compliment all effort/progress toward self-care management. A hug or hand gently placed on the shoulder will impart nurturance.

Motivation comes from a creative spark, a need or desire. Engaging the senior's personal interests within the daily routine will enhance motivation and result in quality of life. Force is never the correct approach to impose upon the senior in any task or self-care activity. The client's unwillingness to follow through with activities within his/her skill level may be a sign of evolving decline or possibly just a low-energy day.

Establishing Trust and Building a Working Relationship

The privilege of working in a senior's home as a private caregiver is one that is earned. The caregiver is working with the senior *and the family*. It is necessary to establish a working relationship with all members of this group with the priority of senior care as the main focus. The elder person has to feel secure with the caregiver and the home situation that is established. To create that security, the senior's ideas must be included in the routine design.

Another important component in the caregiving process is trust. Trust is the foundation upon which all caregiving efforts are based. Trust is earned through dependability and confidentiality. Client and family information remains private. The caregiver who arrives for scheduled visits on time and follows through with designated responsibilities will gain trust.

One of the best ways to establish a comfort zone with the client is to maintain a sense of empathy and humor. Empathy is appreciating the situation from the senior's point of view. An example of empathy is as follows. A senior with diabetes required assistance to bring blood flow to the fingers to check her glucose levels. It was difficult watching her stab several times some mornings to get her blood glucose reading. The caregiver began a fun activity to shake arms down and warm hands with hot towels to make this process less painful.

Humor can help on a low-energy day. Seniors who do not like exercising can laugh at the caregiver who demonstrates exaggerated moves in the routine. The senior gets a show at the caregiver's expense, yet may be motivated to do the exercise routine. Pace the activities based upon the senior's stamina; ask if there is pain or discomfort. If the senior is overworked at any time, he/she will not want to exercise in the future.

For the senior who has difficulty hearing or understanding instructions, the caregiver must communicate clearly and assertively. Express instructions in a clear, slow, and concise manner. Look directly at the senior as you speak. The instruction process needs to be presented at the senior's level of understanding, but not in a patronizing manner. Make sure the client comprehends what is asked of him/her. Have the senior demonstrate the task instructed, to assure clarity.

For the senior living alone, write out brief reminders such as BRUSH TEETH or DRINK WATER. Glue pictures from recycled greeting cards or magazine images on these notes to make them less clinical. Place these notes where the senior will see them.

Bring the senior's interests into the day-to-day process. Discover your client's personal aspects of inspiration through conversation. Find out the type of music the senior likes. The addition of music to the task process can be calming or invigorating based on the atmosphere required. Reading will enrich the senior's life especially for one who has a loss of vision. A favorite meal stimulates the sense of smell and taste. These embellishments added to the caregiving process can be comforting.

Natural aromas from essential oils (non-chemical) are calming and refreshing. In general, women like lavender essential oil, men like clary sage. The essence of grapefruit, orange or lemon, are stimulating and increase energy. Rose essential oil is emotionally soothing. Add these aromas to the bathing process to invigorate and motivate engagement in the task. Bring samples of essential oils to find the most compatible and soothing to the senior.

One senior enjoyed the birds feeding in her backyard. The window that overlooked the feeder was a distance from her usual sitting room. The caregiver created an interest in watching the birds to get the senior to walk a greater distance in the house.

The daughter of a gentleman diagnosed with Alzheimer's disease presented a box of tools he used throughout his career. The discussion that followed was intimate. He was thrilled to connect with the memories that resulted from observing and holding the tools again. She followed up with various boxes that held items of interest from his life. This approach is personalized and enriches the recipient cognitively and emotionally.

A caregiver engaged her client in the activity of singing with guitar accompaniment. Music pages with lyrics were provided. This became an invigorating and motivating occupation. The songs presented were from the senior's lifetime, related to movies of her era. One day the caregiver tried a new approach. She was able to "call up" the original person who performed the songs from the movies on a smartphone. The senior was thrilled to see these musical movie excerpts in their original form. This was fun and inspiring, while the breathing techniques experienced with singing increased oxygen to the brain.

Keeping a journal is a useful way for seniors to record inspirational ideas and track accomplishments. If there is an interest, encourage the client to write, or record through art or photographs, current events happening in his/her life. If the senior is not able to write easily, journaling can take the form of documentation through a picture scrap book process or art portfolio. This may be the best and most concrete way for the senior to record their accomplishments and trigger memories and a warm connection to the current life situation. Add dates and time of events.

Art Portfolio

Make an activity of gathering important items of sentiment the senior chooses. These can include newspaper clippings from articles about family members, loose photographs, poems or artwork the senior created, or letters, greeting cards. The items can relate to family, friends, and pets past and present. Gather any artwork the senior does in day-to-day activity sessions. Organize and date these. Work with the senior to sort, organize and place the selected items into recycled binders or scrapbook-style albums. Decorate with colorful paper. Engage the senior to sign and date all original artwork and possibly write about the art piece. These albums may be stored in a box. Some articles may be chosen for framing and put on display.

The purpose of this activity is to place significant value on precious items representing the senior's life. This process engages planning skills, self-direction and memory in relation to current daily activities. This gives concrete evidence of a lifetime of human relationships.

Ask family members before starting this project. Some items, such as photographs, may be one-of-a-kind and would not be included in the activity to prevent possible loss or damage.

One senior I know had a birthday card loosely stored in a box given to her from her parents on her sixteenth birthday. How this remained intact through the years is unknown. It validates that some seniors have gems that are worth storing in safe keeping for generations to come.

These examples present possible ways to interact with the senior on his/her level of interest. Any extra effort a caregiver puts into the process will help to build a trusting relationship and enhance quality of life for the senior. This type of engagement will help to strengthen the structure of the daily routine and aid the senior's memory in self-care activities. When the senior completes tasks, provide a compliment regarding his/her skills. One senior heard a compliment from her caregiver and was surprised, compliments were given infrequently. The senior responded saying: "That means a lot coming from you."

Chapter 6

Accessibility and Safety in the Home

THE SENIOR'S LIVING ENVIRONMENT MUST BE ADAPTED to assure that he/she is able to manage daily tasks safely. Consistent cleanliness, clutter management, and organization will decrease the potential for accidents or loss of important items. For a senior there are many obstacles that may impede accessibility. Seniors with poor strength will have difficulty opening food containers. Low vision or balance problems will limit one's ability to maneuver through the living space. General weakness will create difficulty in rising from bed, chair or toilet, as well as lifting items from high or low cupboards. The priority must be a clean, safe environment where the layout accommodates the needs of the senior and supports the caregiving team in the process. Once the home is organized for safety, the floor plan must not be changed. Do not move furniture; be sure to put items back if moved while cleaning. Keep frequently used items stored in the same place. This will become the senior's "mental map" of his/her living quarters. This is essential for a senior with low vision/blindness, physical or cognitive losses, and general weakness. Engage the senior in organizing the living space. Respect and maintain his/her wishes within safety allowances.

The home healthcare providers will recommend various types of adaptive equipment and safety grab bars throughout the decline process. These items will assist the senior in ambulation (walking), toilet transfers, bathing and other activities of daily living. The caregiver and family can ask the home healthcare providers for instructions in the correct use of adaptive equipment to assure safety and consistency in caregiving.

Accessibility

The following information indicates areas in the home where accessibility may be compromised. The family will make adjustments in the home with this list as a guide.

› Timed safety lighting and easy reach lights in reading, activity areas, bed/bath
› Easy access to thermostat/climate controls
› Ability to access/use communications devices and telephone.
› Ability to access clothing, manage dresser drawers, closets, reach hangers
› Ability to reach items from cupboards, refrigerator, tools to open containers
› Ability to safely reach/lift cooking items pots/pans
› Access to towels and cosmetics grooming/hygiene supplies in bathroom
› Access to medications and health supplies
› Ambulate in/out of the house safely (fire exits; escape plan required for all levels)

Consult with home healthcare providers for assessment and advice regarding these accessibility needs

› Safe use of stove top; open/close oven, lift items in/out of oven
› Use of kitchen tools or knives
› Bathroom safety grab bars, tub/toilet seat recommendations
› Move from chair/bed to commode
› Safe mobility in bedroom and general living areas; safe sturdy chairs/furniture
› Use of dishwasher or washer/dryer and safe return of items into storage
› Driving safety
› Transfer in/out of the car

Any adaptations arranged for the senior must be respected and maintained for safe navigation or easy reach of needed items. Seasonal changes will require preparation for lighting variations and clothing requirements. Snow removal for accessibility will be necessary in some areas

Accessibility includes the senior's ability to communicate using a phone. Several phones will need to be placed at key locations for the senior to access. It is recommended that a large-print communications board is placed near the phone with a list of essential phone numbers to help the senior access help or assistance. If the senior is skilled in using programmed phone numbers, set up the phone in a manner that is easy for the senior to speedily contact family and friends.

Practice the steps for phone use frequently with the senior to help maintain the required skill. A senior with a hearing impairment will need a lighted/vibrating phone with speaker boost.

Medical safety alert systems are important ways to access emergency help and provide peace of mind for the senior, family members and caregivers at times when the senior is alone. This is essential for a senior at level 2 waning into level 3, living alone. The senior will need to practice the use of medical alert systems. Review often with the senior how and when to use this device. It may become a forgotten tool if the senior has intermittent memory loss, even if he/she is wearing an alert button.

Computers allow additional means of communicating or accessing information through e-mail and the internet. A senior who is able to use a computer should be encouraged to maintain this skill and enjoy the social and educational connections the computer offers.

Accessibility Adaptations for Particular Rooms

The following section lists changes that will be needed to adapt the home for safety. Some recommendations are advised for all functioning levels as indicated. It is recommended that consultation with home modifications experts commence prior to installing any structural support systems. Experts can provide specific measurements for architectural changes regarding wheelchair accessibility and installing grab bars that require specific measurements for the individual senior's height.

Easy access to light switches with bright lighting is essential at every entrance, in every room, hallway and closet/storage space. Lighting is necessary in the kitchen, at common work areas, as well as at side tables where the senior sits. Place emergency flashlights at easy-to-reach locations.

Entranceways

Seniors at all functional levels
> Wide exterior entrance area (preferably 36 inches) no clutter; no throw rugs.
> If the entrance room permits, a boot/shoe tray may be placed off to the side of the walkway, or just inside of the closet. Provide a seat to use when donning outside shoes/boots.

Seniors using a walker
› A smooth flat surface or inclined ramp to the car will provide safe accessibility.
› All inside entrances require clear wide path to accommodate door space.

Seniors using a wheelchair
› A smooth flat surface or inclined ramp to the car will be required.
› When pushing a client in a wheelchair up or down a ramp, always keep the back of the chair toward the downward incline. See illustration at the end of this chapter.
› Entrance threshold requires smooth floor board weather stripping (minimal threshold step: one-half-inch beveled or one-quarter-inch square) as well as clear wide path.
› Inside doorways need to be 36 inches wide.
› Entrance coat closet requires low hanging bar for accessibility.
› If a closet is not available, a lowered hanging rack or shortened hall tree will work.
› A hanger with a cloth bag secured will store hats/gloves/scarves within reach.
› For ease in mobilizing the wheelchair have plastic floor runners placed in the navigational areas of the house. Check office supply/equipment resources for isle runners with non-slip bottom. This is needed only in rooms with wall-to-wall carpeting.

Bathrooms

Seniors at all functional levels
› Grab bars at the toilet and in the shower are recommended as an early intervention.
› *Monitor water temperature setting at the water heater* to prevent accidental burns.
› Toiletry items have easy access when placed in covered baskets on the counter top.
› Store towels/wash cloths where the senior can reach them.
› Keep loose towels off the floor to prevent falls. Towels hung on towel bars may be secured with a rubber band. Fold the hand towel over the bar, hold the two layers of the towel together under the bar and pull a rubber band around both layers. Slide the rubber band up toward the bar to allow the two ends of the towel to hang to dry hands.

Seniors using a walker

> In a small bathroom, if space does not allow for the walker, direct the senior to hold on to the counters and grab bars for support in walking.
> A raised toilet seat with grab bars will be needed.
> A shower seat with grab bars on the walls of the shower stall or within the tub area are essential, plus a bath mat.
> The senior's feet need to be touching the ground with a raised toilet or shower seat. This will assure safe ability to rise from seat.

Seniors using a wheelchair

> Expand entrance space with a pocket door if needed.
> Room for assisted transfer between wheelchair and toilet/shower seat is essential if the senior is not strong enough to stand and transfer independently.
> A hydraulic lift may be required for safe bathing transfers.
> In a small bathroom, if space does not allow for the wheelchair, a commode chair will need to be placed where it is accessible in a private area outside of the bathroom. Also sponge bathing will commence. Home healthcare providers will instruct in these circumstances.

Kitchens

Safety in the kitchen includes handling of stove and hot items; the use of cutting tools or food processing appliances. Safe food handling and proper storage are included in a basic ADL task evaluation. The home healthcare providers will determine the senior's ability to safely manage meal preparation and kitchen responsibilities.

Seniors at all functioning levels

> The cooking items used by the senior are placed in priority areas for easy access.
> Cooking for one or two can be done with smaller pots/pans.
> Remove kitchen items no longer used, or too awkward for the senior to handle.
> The refrigerator must be set up with shelves designated for the senior's easy reach.
> Any items the senior will lift in/out of refrigerator must be light enough for safe handling without spillage or dropping.
> Refrigerator door must open to a counter top for easy placement of items removed from the fridge.
> Food storage containers must be easy to open with tools available to assist.

> Pot holders for handling hot items must be available at micro-wave and stove/oven.
> Counter space must be available next to stove top, microwave or oven for easy placement of hot foods.
> Kitchen towels may be secured to towel racks with rubber band or button loop.
> Clean out the toaster frequently, crumbs/raisins may become a fire hazard
> Limit or eliminate breakable glass containers.
> Secure sharp knives in a safe location.

Seniors using a walker
> All areas of the kitchen used must remain open and clear for ambulation.
> Limit the type and amount of items carried on the seat platform of a walker.
> Use countertops to move items from one place to another.

Seniors using a wheelchair
> Counters/sink must be lowered with open leg space below.
> Appliances such as microwave, stove top must be lowered for easy reach.
> Dishes, silverware, kitchen tools must be lowered to accessible storage cabinets and/or drawers.

Bedrooms

Seniors at all functional levels
> Bed bars are essential for transfers in/out of the bed if the senior has compromised strength. Or a medical bed may be considered for those functioning at level 3.
> Plastic mattress covers are recommended for incontinence.
> Clothing may be hung in the closet, or placed in dresser drawers if the senior is able to open them, or openly visible/accessible on a counter top.
> Be sure all clothing is fitted correctly: too big may create trip possibility.
> Bedding must not hang down to the floor.
> Remove dusters and extra pillows as they may become a trip/fall hazard if left loosely on or around the bed.
> No throw rugs on the floor and no clutter to impede ambulation.
> A bedside commode may be needed for toilet access through the night. A caregiver or family member must schedule time

daily to empty the commode.

› A bedside table will hold all essential items with a wastepaper basket nearby.

Seniors using a walker

› Space must remain open for clear ambulation and easy access to commode chair and personal items in closet or storage compartments.

› Grab bars on the bed will assist with transfers in and out.

Seniors using a wheelchair

› A closet with clear floor space and lowered hanging bars is recommended.

› Access and transfer accommodations for bed and bedside commode must be available.

Safety

Ramp Safety When Using a Wheelchair

When ambulating or pushing a wheelchair up or down a ramp, always keep the open seat of the chair facing the top of the ramp to prevent falling. Figures 1 and 2.

Ramp designs are recommended to measure 1 inch rise for every 12 inches in length.

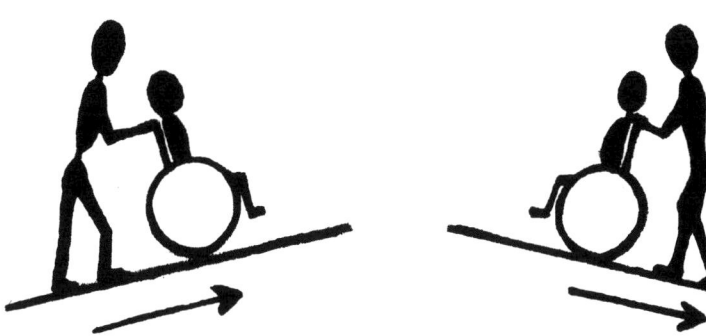

Fig. 1. Up the ramp   Fig. 2. Down the ramp

Housekeeping and Storage for Safe/Easy Accessibility

Family members and caregiver(s) need to take responsibility regarding the accessibility of important items. It is vital that all commonly used items (by the senior and caregiving team) are consistently placed in specific storage areas within easy reach. The following tips identify items that both the senior and caregivers will need to access.

› Medication packs need to be accessible yet safely stored out of the reach of children or seniors who are unable to manage the medication routine.
› Place heavy items such as milk in small containers to assist access for the senior.
› Keep refrigerator clean with wholesome foods available, in easy-to-open containers, date food items that are easily perishable.
› Place shampoo in small plastic containers.
› Keep supplies for incontinence available near the toilet or commode chair with discard basket nearby.
› Be sure toilet paper and facial tissues are available where needed.
› If possible, remove wall-to-wall carpeting and replace with an easy-to-clean floor. This is helpful mainly in the senior's toilet areas and frequent living areas. It improves wheelchair or walker accessibility as well.
› Frequent housecleaning will be needed to sanitize kitchen, bathroom and living spaces. Provide orientation to the hired housekeeper or caregiver regarding the correct storage process for cleaning products. Stress that items must be kept in assigned areas for safety and easy accessibility.
› Always replace any items or furniture moved in the cleaning process, or as visitors arrive and utilize the senior's living space.
› Be sure all phones throughout the house are working properly and within easy reach.
› Keep plenty of drinking water available at chair side, bedside, and dinner table to improve hydration.

Preparing for the Job

A clean, accessible environment begins with tools and supplies available for the job. The personal health of the caregiver and senior must be regarded as services are rendered in terms of preventing cross-contamination. The caregiver who is prepared for the job should bring a dust mask, sterile gloves, cleaning gloves, non-skid, in-home work shoes, and cover garments. These items, except the shoes/cover garments, may be purchased by the family and made available in the senior's home.

Housekeeping Tips

In the process of housecleaning, the caregiver/housekeeper is advised to wear a dust mask, cleaning gloves and cover garments. When assisting the senior in ADL's, such as bathing, grooming and hygiene tasks, the caregiver will wear sterile gloves. Keep finger nails trimmed short to prevent scratching when helping with personal care, such as dressing. Wash hands with soap and water as you enter the home and as you leave.

› Use protective gloves and dust mask for all cleaning tasks.
› Wear in-house shoes with non-slip soles, not street shoes.
› Use environmentally safe cleaners such as white vinegar, washing soda, or other "green" products.
› Follow the senior's suggestions about his/her special cleaning techniques.
› Follow the senior's guide in how to manage laundry.
› Sanitize kitchen and bathroom as a priority; use disinfectants as needed.
› Sanitize at each visit: kitchen counter tops, cutting boards, table surface, and sink.
› Have specific dedicated cleaning rags to prevent cross contamination.
› Sanitize cleaning rags and buckets and mops after use.
› Clean the following surfaces regularly: commode chair, walker, cane, grab bars, and wheelchair.
› Bring in fresh air to eliminate odors; avoid chemical air fresheners.
› Request tools and supplies needed from the family.
› Do not use cleaning rags or tools that have been used in other residences.
› Read container labels for poison or chemical storage instructions. Even some cleaning supplies are dangerous. Store properly. Place potentially dangerous items in a box away from the senior's reach and discuss the removal process with the family.
› Bring attention to anything that is broken; this is to deflect possible blame later. If you (as a housekeeper/caregiver) break something, call attention to the accident immediately and offer to pay for the damage.

The caregiver should always be clean, presentable, and ready for services. A neat personal appearance will result in trust and respect from the senior and family.

Clearing Clutter

Clutter management and consistent organization are necessary to prevent safety hazards. Establish a means of sorting what comes into the house: recycle, throw away, file, store. Recycling may be connected with the house-keeping routine to insure an outward flow of items. Talk with family members and the senior before throwing anything away and agree upon the best storage places to contain items.

> Recycling helps in removing surplus items.
> Schedule time to organizing table tops, counters, and other sur-faces where items collect, as well as, storage closets, kitchen pantry shelves.
> Keep like items in the designated area where they will be used.
> Place out-of-season clothing/bedding into storage.

Consistent organization is helpful to make the senior's living area clean and clutter free. This is the cornerstone for home safety and accessibility. It is imperative to discuss with the senior and family contact person the best way to remove clutter or discard items. Do not throw away any items with-out permission. Items that may seem unimportant to the caregiver could have sentimental or unexpected value to the senior or family members.

Chapter 7

Balance and Ambulation

BALANCE AND ITS EFFECT ON THE SENIOR'S ABILITY TO WALK (ambulate) will be evaluated by the home healthcare providers. The senior will present with one of various possible levels of need. The home healthcare providers will determine which adaptive device is required, if any. The following list shows the continuum of decline in balance and ambulation.

› Independent – walking without assistance
› Minimum level of assistance – walking with a cane
› Medium level of assistance – walking with a walker
› Those unable to ambulate on their own require a wheelchair or automated appliance

The caregiver remains on the weaker side of the senior for assistance or stand-by assistance in all of the above levels. Senior and caregiver must wear shoes or slippers with non-slip soles while ambulating. The walker or cane will need to be adjusted by a therapist from the home healthcare provider's team to fit the senior's height and weight.

Wheelchair ambulation presents a greater need for accessibility modification including a ramp at entrance. Also, if the senior is unable to transfer due to inability to bear weight, large adaptive equipment will be needed, such as, a lift to move in/out of bed or shower, with assistance. Home healthcare providers or a *rehabilitation consultant* with specific training in *home modifications* will recommend the required home adaptations as indicated by the individual needs of the senior. The family and caregiver(s) will need training specific to one in a wheelchair and the adaptive equipment recommended.

Fall Prevention and Safety Checklist

The following information will serve as a guideline for the caregiver and family. Extra vigilance must be used as visitors may move items or even furniture in the house as they occasionally drop by.

> › Keep the home clutter free inside and out; snow removed from entrances in winter.
> › Secure electronic cords away from walking areas; coil and wrap with twist tie.
> › Remove all throw rugs; secure the edges of thick carpets down on floors and stairs.
> › Keep frequently used items at easy reach in kitchen, bathroom, bedroom, living room.
> › Have security lights set to turn on automatically; light switches within easy reach.
> › Have an emergency generator turn on automatically if electricity goes out.
> › Use night lights in bathroom, hallways and bedroom.
> › Add railings to both sides of all stairways. Block stairways that are not in use.
> › Use strong leg first when walking up a stairway and weak leg first when walking down.
> › Railings may be placed throughout the house as needed in the most used areas.
> › Use walker, cane, wheelchair safely per home healthcare provider instructions.
> › Begin each day donning shoes or house slippers with non-slip soles for safe walking.
> › Don shoes or slippers in seated position.
> › Be sure the senior has solid chairs with arms to sit and rise safely.
> › The senior must use proper sitting techniques to sit and rise from a chair.

Sitting/Rising from the Chair

Use these verbal instructions to help seniors sit or rise from a chair in a safe manner.

To sit: back up to the chair until you feel the seat at the back of your legs (Fig. 3). Bring hands back to grasp arms of the chair (Fig. 4). Slowly sit using arms of the chair (Fig. 5).

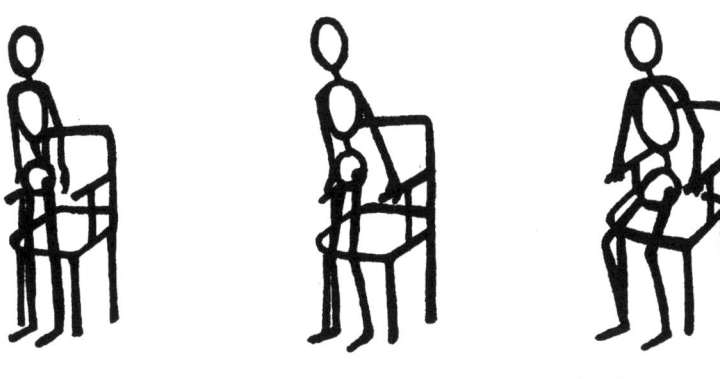

Fig. 3.   Fig. 4.   Fig. 5.

To rise: Grasp arms of the chair and move forward in the chair (Fig. 6). Use the arms of the chair and abdominal/leg muscles to lift to standing position (Fig. 7 and Fig. 8).

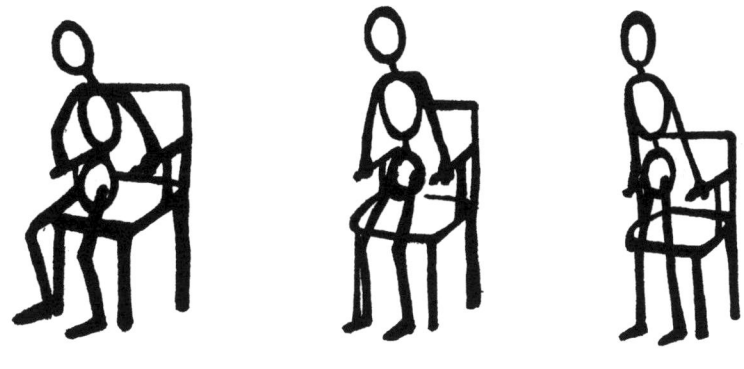

Fig. 6.   Fig. 7.   Fig. 8.

To sit in a chair *while using a walker,* back up to the chair, lock the walker before sitting in the chair. Direct the senior to *use the arms of the chair to sit and rise, not the walker.*

For a walker designated as *safe for sitting, the senior must always lock the walker both before sitting and when rising.*

Chapter 8

Body Mechanics and Posture Alignment

CARING FOR THE ELDERLY is difficult work and requires physical strength. *Body mechanics,* the correct use of our muscles in coordination with the pull of gravity, will assist the caregiver who needs to lift items like groceries, clean around and under large furniture pieces and assist the senior in and out of a chair or bed, or on and off the toilet. The practice of correct body mechanics outlined in this chapter is directed toward the caregiver and family members to prevent injury on the job. This chapter also exemplifies posture alignment for a comfortable approach to tasks in which the senior may engage.

Responding to Gravity

The body responds to gravity in two ways: (1) We *consciously* use the abdominal muscles to maintain an upright posture; and (2) We maintain balance within the pull of gravity *subconsciously,* through an automatic reflexive response in the inner ear. *The inner ear contains the vestibular system that supports an upright posture through the head-righting reflex.*

Simply stated: The inner ear works reflexively, automatically without conscious effort, to prevent falls. Correct posture, *maintained consciously,* supports this automatic process. Maintaining correct posture in combination with the vestibular system is the key to safe body mechanics and the foundation of injury prevention. The coordinated effort between balance and posture allows smooth movement when walking, standing, or sitting. This also helps stabilize the body's trunk while lifting heavy items or when transferring a senior from chair to commode.

The abdominal muscles are structured to hold the trunk of the body in an upright vertical position on a long-term basis. The abdominal muscles are designed, physiologically, to remain in contraction for extended lengths of time. However, it takes conscientious practice to remind our abdominal muscles to do this job. Correct posture creates core stability and structural support as our arms and hands complete the task with the least amount of energy expenditure. Practicing correct posture also decreases the chance of joint injury as it places the body in proper alignment.

Ways to Support Correct Posture and Joint Alignment

The following tips will help to prevent injury for both the senior and caregiver.

> Use abdominal muscles to extend the trunk upward. This will eliminate weight from lower back (lumbar area) and neck (cervical area). See pelvis tilt illustration on the next page.
> Remind the senior to use abdominal muscles to extend the trunk upward while walking, while in a seated position, or when rising from a chair.
> Use heel-to-toe foot placement with toes pointed forward while walking to prevent misalignment at hips/knees.
> Do not lock knees while walking or standing.
> Support the lower back (lumbar) with a pillow while the senior is seated upright, or in a wheelchair. Lumbar support is required while working at a table, desk or a computer.

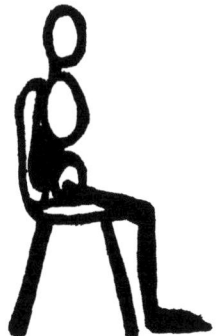

Fig. 9. Lumbar support while seated

Posture Review

Balance works reflexively; thinking is not involved. Posture, however, must be maintained conscientiously. If we do not maintain correct upright posture, the reflexive response of the inner ear will be to adjust the head to compensate. This adjustment misaligns the neck and shoulders. Over time this creates kyphosis or a hunchback. Also the lower back will suffer strain due to the weight of the trunk misplaced in a forward position.

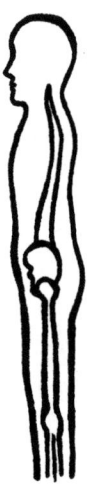 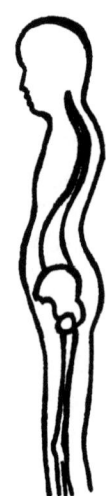

Fig. 10. Correct posture: pelvis in upright position

Fig. 11. Incorrect posture: pelvis tilted forward

The abdominal muscles must hold the pelvis in an upright vertical position to maintain correct spinal alignment.

Proper Position for Lifting

The box drawn around the three figures below represents the safety parameters and position for injury prevention while lifting. The illustrated box outlines the limits where one must maintain the body to remain safely inside of the base of gravity. The base of gravity is a specific area beneath us that allows the gravitational force to assist us through movement as it prevents injury or falls. In other words, any movement outside of this base, such as a tilt, over-reach, or stumble, may end in a fall.

Position dolly or cart close to the item. Approach heavy item directly in front. Keep the item you are about to lift close to your body. Place the feet directly under the widest area of the hips. Use the abdominal and leg muscles to stand and lift simultaneously. Get help if the item is awkward or too heavy to lift within base of gravity.

Begin in a squat position; use the abdominal muscles to keep the pelvis and back extended in an upright position (Fig. 12). Grasp item, hold close to the body within the gravitational base, not extended outward (Fig. 13). Use leg and abdominal muscles to rise from a squat to standing position (Fig. 14).

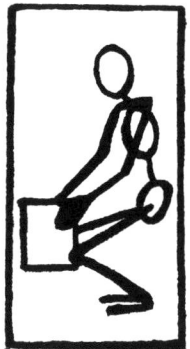 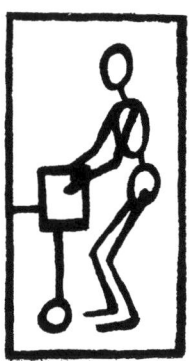 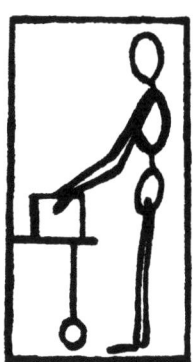

Fig. 12. Base of gravity within box

Fig. 13. Grasp and lift

Fig. 14. Place item on cart

The base of gravity, as illustrated within the box, also applies to movement such as sitting/rising from a chair. Imagine this box around the senior as she/he sits or rises from a chair. Any tilting outside of the base of gravity will indicate instability. Support the senior on the weaker side if he /she is unstable.

Transferring from a Chair to a Commode

Lifting a senior for transfer, in/out of chair, bed, or on/off toilet, requires training from the home healthcare providers: a physical therapist (PT) or occupational therapist (OT). Do not try to transfer a client without hands-on instructions from an OT or PT. *The following illustrations are to be used as a reminder to assure proper body mechanics, after one receives training in this process.* Transferring a client is required only for those who are able to bear weight on his/her legs, yet are too weak to rise from a chair independently.

Both the senior and the caregiver must wear solid shoes with non-slip soles. Place a commode chair or wheelchair perpendicular to the chair in which the senior sits. Put the gait belt on at the waistline and tighten until snug but not uncomfortable. Instruct the senior to place feet firmly on the ground and point them forward as much as possible. The caregiver stands in front of the senior with his or her feet placed in front of the senior's feet.

Caregiver begins in a shallow squat position, using the abdominal muscles to keep trunk extended in an upright position (see Fig. 15). Instruct senior to place his/her arms on the arms of the chair. Caregiver holds the gait belt firmly and instructs the senior on the count of three to rise together (Fig. 16). Caregiver uses leg and abdominal muscles to rise from squat position to standing while, simultaneously, bringing the senior to a standing position (Fig. 17).

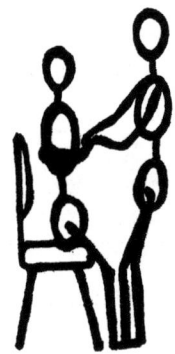 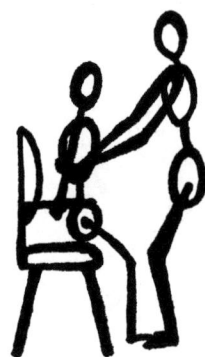 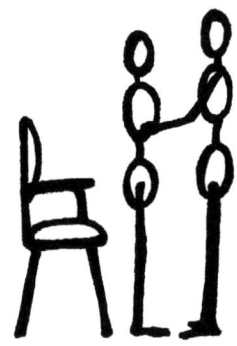

Fig. 15. Base of gravity within box   Fig. 16. Grasp gait belt   Fig. 17. Lift

Caregiver instructs the senior to pivot toward the commode or wheel chair (Fig. 18). The senior sits on the commode chair or wheelchair (Fig. 19).

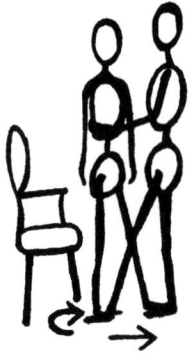 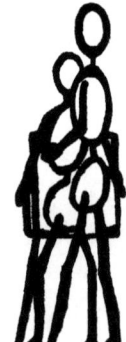

Fig. 18. Pivot to commode   Fig. 19. Squat to sit

Body Mechanics for Fine Motor Tasks

Fine motor tasks are activities we do with our hands and arms while seated or standing at a counter. The muscles of our hands, arms and shoulders are not designed to be in continuous use for long periods of time. These muscles are physiologically designed differently than the weight bearing, muscles of the legs and abdomen. Frequent rest and pacing will prevent fatigue and injury. Rest breaks should be every twenty to thirty minutes for the elderly. For example, seniors who hold the handles of the walker for extended periods of time should take a rest at regular, paced intervals. The same is true for anyone using a computer for long periods of time.

Task preparation is a safe way to begin any activity. Work at a surface that is comfortable. The height of counter top surfaces need to be at least thirty-six inches if standing. Taller people may want the counter higher. If shoulders have to be raised to work at the surface, it is too high. If one needs to bend to reach the countertop, it is too low. If working at a table, the height should be between thirty and thirty-two inches.

Gather tools and items needed before beginning a task. Follow safety precautions when using sharp tools. Be sure to wear a dust mask if a job presents dust particles or exposes one to chemicals such as paint or cleaning supplies.

It is easy to forget our posture as we become involved in a table-top task, or as we stand at a counter. These activities will require vigilance to correct posture and frequent rest breaks to prevent over-use of small muscles and joints. The following suggestions are helpful.

› Use abdominal muscles to extend the trunk and to correct posture frequently.

› Use lower back support for any seated task, or for one in a wheelchair: place a small pillow at the lumbar curve of the spine.

› Do not hold items in one hand for extended amounts of time. This is called static hold. For example, set a paint can down rather than hold it while painting. Use a book holder to support the book for hands-free reading.

› Ask for assistance if a task is too difficult to manage alone.

› Take frequent breaks from tasks that keep body in same position long lengths of time.

› Pace yourself, respect physical limitations in any task; practice deep breathing, often.

› Take steps of a task in paced increments. Plan enough time to allow for stretch breaks, toilet breaks and intake of nutrition and water.

› If seated in a wheelchair, one must shift weight frequently, every 15 to 30 minutes, to prevent pressure sores.

› Use non-dominant to assist dominant hand.

› Take breaks while using a walker. If balance allows, release hands from the handles one at a time to relieve static hold.

Energy Conservation

For the caregiver, family members or seniors who work in a personal office, the following tips will provide energy conservation.

› Take frequent breaks when using the computer or hand held electronic device; release the mouse or electronic device to stretch and relax the hands.

› Use an ergonomic computer chair to ensure proper lower back support in the lumbar area.

› Hold phone to the ear no longer than ten minutes at a time; use speaker mode whenever possible.

› Stand and stretch often; hold stretches for twenty to thirty seconds or longer. This is important for one watching TV for long movies or extended periods of time.

Energy conservation guidelines for those who work in food preparation and manage kitchen tasks are as follows.

› When cooking, use low to medium heat to be able to control the process with less stress.

› Chop foods in seated position ahead of dinner preparation time.

› Sit while engaging in fine motor tasks. Use a stool at the kitchen counter, or for the senior with balance problems, a chair at the kitchen table.

› Do not push beyond the limits of energy resources. Those with arthritis should work no more than twenty to thirty minutes at a time to reduce stress on joints.

› Clean up after each task; return tools and supplies to a well-organized storage place.

It is recommended that anyone in the role of caregiver keep fit physically and mindfully put these important body mechanics into practice. The caregiver who follows these suggestions will prevent personal injury. Also these tips will enhance the guidance of the senior, with safety as a priority, in task management.

Chapter 9

Range-of-Motion and Exercise

JOINT FLEXIBILITY DIMINISHES as we age or with disuse. Joint range-of-motion (ROM) is the ability to flex (bend) or extend (straighten) a joint through its full measure of movement. Healthy joints not used on a regular basis may exhibit decreased ROM. Seniors with limited ROM will have difficulty performing ADL's independently. Conversely, seniors who consistently manage ADL's as independently as possible, will maintain joint flexibility. Exercise and active engagement in self-care will help to prevent a loss of ROM.

The movement/range in which one moves the joints on his/her own, without assistance, is called active range-of-motion (AROM). Examples include raising one's arms to pull a shirt on over the head. The arms are extended up and flex to pull the shirt down around the back. Also included in this action is flexion and extension at the neck plus wrist and hand motions. To dress the lower limb in a seated position, one must bend at the trunk; flex legs at the knees and hips to pull pants over the feet. Then a standing position will extend the trunk to pull the pants up. This demonstrates the importance of allowing the senior to dress/undress as independently as possible. This is a good daily workout.

One complication found in those who are inactive is the *predominance of a natural reflex pattern* that promotes flexion of all joints. This flexion pattern can be seen in fingers curling to a closed position, or the spinal column curling into a hunchbacked (kyphosis) position. This curling process will lead to contractures. A contracture is the inability to move a joint through full ROM due to shortening of the tendons or muscles around the joint.

Contractures are caused by inactivity, prolonged joint misalignment, or joint structure breakdown resulting from arthritis or injuries sustained earlier in life. Contractures become permanent and do not allow the normal, full ROM, even with a regular exercise routine. Nonetheless, even in cases of decreased flexibility, joints should be exercised through whatever ROM still remains. The senior can engage in gentle stretch activities that extend the spinal column, arms, hands, legs and feet to counteract contractures and the natural flexion reflex pattern.

A senior who has had a knee or hip or shoulder replacement will have an individualized plan designed by the home healthcare providers suited for one following surgery. There will be limitations in body positioning. The home healthcare providers will instruct the family and caregiver in safe, specific movement at the involved joints and extremities, as well as limitations in ROM for these individuals.

A caregiver must never manipulate the senior's hands, arms, legs or feet to push beyond the senior's AROM. This will cause injury. Unless a caregiver has had hands-on-training in the correct process of assisting one through ROM, it is contraindicated to physically move a person's extremities for increased ROM.

In summary, ROM exercises for each individual senior must be discussed with the home healthcare providers who will provide general active range-of-motion exercises that the senior will be able to do independently. With this plan included in the day-to-day activities, it will be easy to maintain the senior's current range-of-motion, as well as stamina to complete daily tasks.

Walking Is the Best and Easiest Exercise

In addition to ROM, exercise is an important part of the senior's daily routine. The home healthcare providers will instruct the family and caregiver in safe, specific exercises for each individual senior. With the guidance of the home healthcare providers, the caregiver or family members, will be able to engage the senior in specific recommended exercises on a routine basis. Occupational therapists and physical therapists will provide written, illustrated handouts indicating the correct exercise plan for each senior individually. Follow these exercises as specified.

One exercise that should be part of the senior's routine is walking.

Walking is the easiest, most effective way to improve our physical well-being. Walking helps to organize our thinking (Hopkins and Smith 1978, 134–140). The act of walking engages right/left stepping, arms swinging naturally, vision expanding. The whole body is engaged in physical action. This initiates balance and protective reflex mechanisms as our body moves in space in relation to gravity and environmental surroundings. Through a walking program, coordination plus overall strength, agility and balance improve. This must be paced and not exhaustive.

Prior to walking, practice stretching to extend the spinal column, legs, feet, arms, hands and fingers. The senior can engage in stretching in bed before rising, or in a seated position. Do not lock knees during stretch exercises or while walking.

To maintain proper body alignment and posture while walking, the abdominal muscles must be used to hold the trunk in an extended upright position. Toes should be pointed forward. This will ease the lower back and assist the hips and knees in weight bearing during the activity.

Engage the senior at levels 2 and 3 in regular walking activities throughout the house or outside if balance and stability allow. Ask the home healthcare providers for advice on outside ambulation specific to the senior.

Deep breathing is an important component of all activities. This brings oxygen to the muscles and brain and supports cognitive functioning. Frequently remind the senior to breath during exercises and regular activities. Five minutes of simple breathing in and out is refreshing. Exercises like singing or practicing deep breathing will bring a burst of oxygen to the brain and body. Check frequently for lightheadedness. Practice these breathing exercises in a seated position.

Exercises for Seniors Functioning at Level 1

For seniors who are independent, a more vigorous exercise routine may become part of his/her lifestyle. Some current methods of exercise include physical and cognitive components. Dance, swimming, Tai Chi and yoga are examples. The combined cognitive and physical effort required to learn these procedural routines challenge the performer in body and mind. The whole-body workout derived from practicing these ancient activities contributes to increased energy, improved balance, muscle tone, flexibility and mental clarity. When one engages this type of exercise on a regular basis, the decline process of aging may be minimized. A doctor's approval must be attained for safety assurance before engaging in any exercise program.

Chapter 10

Professional Performance

ANYONE WHO WISHES TO PROVIDE IN-HOME SERVICES for the elderly must consider the characteristics of a supportive caregiver as outlined in Chapter 1, "The Aging Process." This will help one to determine if she/he has the personality for the job. Also the following information offers tips to assure success in the day-to-day tasks of care provision.

Confidentiality

Once the caregiver is hired, the senior and family members become clients. The privacy of each client is the cornerstone of professional behavior. All aspects of caregiving, including information about the senior's health and well-being must be kept in confidence and should not become a topic of conversation with anyone. Breaking this rule will result in a loss of trust and possibly dire consequences. Follow these guidelines to insure confidentiality.

> › Do not use the client's name or let anyone know of your caregiving duties.
> › Inform those who know you and your client, mutually, that you will not share information due to confidentiality constraints.
> › Do not discuss family information or share medical information

regarding the client with anyone.

› Do not tell anyone over the phone or at the door the age or health status of the client. This may put them in danger.

› Do not leave phone messages about the client's condition with anyone. Permission must be granted on the agreement for caregiving services to approve recording messages on the phone to the family contact person(s).

› Have a primary and secondary contact person identified in the contract agreement with whom to divulge sensitive information or problems as required.

› Make daily charting available to only those who need to know; store this documentation in a private place.

› Photographs should not be taken of the senior or family members unless permission is granted.

› No personal information or pictures of the senior or family members should ever be posted on social media.

Objectivity

Caregiving that is provided in a neutral, objective manner will offer unobstructed support to the senior and family. Objectivity means observing how the senior engages in his/her daily routine without judgment. The caregiver must become skilled in observation in order to insure objectivity and present facts in an unbiased manner. The senior may try to hide a loss of skills and may claim to have no problems performing various tasks. It is only through the process of observing the senior's actions during task completion that the caregiver will gather key information regarding safety and competence. The caregiver will then be able to cite examples of task steps that the senior found easy or difficult to accomplish. Caregivers should not draw conclusions based upon that which is observed. The importance of observing objectively is to provide information, with examples, to the family and primary care physician regarding the senior's functioning level.

Problem solving with the family follows accurate descriptions of the senior's task process. The caregiver's observations will provide evidence of the need for change if skills are improved or declining.

Communications Skills

Communication is the foundation upon which a relationship is built. The manner in which one communicates will reveal a lot about character as demonstrated in how one expresses ideas tactfully, and listens respectfully.

Working in a team requires tactful communications. Competence in both speaking and listening is needed to bring pertinent information to the group in a timely manner. Sensitive issues need to be discussed at an appropriate time to assure confidentiality and clarity and without disruption. Opposing opinions need to be aired when the safety of the client or anyone in the caregiving role, is at stake. This is not a time to place blame. The focus is safety and client care. Assertive communication with examples of observations, are the structure from which problem solving may happen. Topics of concern that are not within the caregivers training/credentials must be directed to others who have an expertise in these areas to assure correct care provision

Listening

Acquiring a sensitivity to the other person's perspective is gained through listening and accessing his or her point of view. Empathy is respecting or appreciating the feelings of others, even though we may not agree or feel the same. Working within the intimate circle of the elderly and their families creates many experiences that provoke an extensive range of emotions. As family members and the senior express feelings about end-of-life issues a receptive listener will be appreciated.

There are times when the senior is not fully respected and his/her message is minimized. This may lead to health complications and accidents. Some seniors are used to this type of treatment and will not express thoughts or feelings freely. Family members and caregivers must not fall into this complacent/passive treatment of the senior team member. The caregiver, family and senior will have to polish and practice listening skills in a patient manner. Ask questions to engage the senior.

The skilled listener will maintain full eye contact and remain quiet as the other person speaks. Turn the television or radio down to reduce external noise when important information is being discussed. The listener will allow the speaker to complete all sentences to assure full reception of what is being announced. A responsive listener will repeat back what was expressed to confirm understanding, and receive the information without judgment. Ask for clarification and check the accuracy with which we heard the contents of the speaker's message. Practice clearing the mind to absorb the speaker's words. Full reception cannot happen without a clear head.

Speaking

Communicating with the family will require a summary of how the senior is doing on a regular basis. Provide facts and observations objectively. Choose words carefully taking into consideration the feelings of other people. Bring truth to the issue as understood at the current time. Withhold judgment. Express your thoughts directly with key points that support the message. If your findings lead you to think that the senior is at a safety risk, in activity performance or with the home environment, give examples of observations.

The use of "I" statements allows us to agree or to voice a difference of opinion, such as "I have observed _____ and feel this activity is unsafe for _____ at this time." We must be tactful and give examples to show why we have a difference of opinion.

If, as a caregiver, you feel the safety of the senior client is in jeopardy and the family is not responsive, fully discuss the senior's safety issues with the contact person providing documented examples. If elder abuse is suspected, the caregiver can make an anonymous call to Adult Protective Services in the local area for information regarding the situation.

The following guidelines are recommended for the caregiver to help foster a neutral relationship with all those interacting in the caregiving process.

> Work with the designated contact person to minimize misunderstandings.
> Alert the contact person of any observed changes or problems as soon as noted.
> Describe observations with examples.
> Document the type of information provided to the contact person and how the information was communicated: phone, text or e-mail.
> Document any instructions given by the contact person and follow up on the intervention.
> Document the actual interventions provided by the caregiver.
> Remain neutral, initiate the plan designated by the contact person and family.
> Do not create conflict; work within the bounds of safety; focus on senior care.
> Pace tasks to conserve the senior's energy. Help the client to maintain basic personal care.
> Keep to an agreed-upon routine as much as possible. Document when and why the senior or others involved may wish to deviate from the usual daily schedule of activities.
> Document any objections the senior expresses to following the Care Plan or recommended activities. The client may not feel well, or the objection may indicate a physical or mental decline if persistent.
> Keep focus on the senior, especially when others are in the

home (visitors or those who may be living in the senior's home). Avoid distractions.

› Caregivers must not talk about personal issues while on paid time. The primary need is to focus on the senior and family members.

Confidentiality, objectivity, and communications skills are important requirements for the hired caregivers. These guidelines will help one polish his/her professional performance.

Caregiver Credentials

The caregiver who provides more than housekeeping will need training in areas of special needs. Classes at a local community college, or evening classes provided through the public school system will be available for further education. Some colleges offer caregiver certification courses. Training in cardio pulmonary resuscitation (CPR) is also recommended. Information regarding this certification may be attained from the local fire department or the county health department.

The caregiver should attain a food handlers card from the local county health department if cooking is a required service for the senior. This is an important credential to attain and list on the caregiver's résumé. The training provided to secure a food handler's card may be as easy as attending a brief one-day seminar. The caregiver will learn how to handle, cook and store food properly, plus the prevention of cross contamination of foods.

Add statements to your résumé reflecting each training experience, class or continuing education seminar when completed. Keep copies of any certificates attained.

Managing the Changing Needs of the Elderly

Changes in senior's needs and living environment will happen over time. Caregiver credentials are an important part of service provision. It is contraindicated to move into levels of care if one is not trained and experienced in those areas. The following three-way plan explains variations in levels of care. Advanced senior care certifications may be obtained through the American Red Cross, the National Association for Home Care and Hospice, or a reputable college for nursing. Check with the Better Business Bureau and local/state or federal agencies for minimum requirements.

Service Plan One

This is a basic level of care which includes housekeeping, companionship, meal preparation, and managing errands or shopping. Formulate hourly wage based upon comparable wages of contractors providing this type of service.

Service Plan Two

This is the medial level of care and may include (along with the tasks listed above), additional services, such as, standby assistance in personal care: dressing/bathing, increased safety monitoring and ADL intervention. Formulate hourly fee with recognition of specific skills/certifications required to attend to personal care needs.

Service Plan Three

This plan increases care intervention and includes skills required for such activities as wheelchair transfers using a special lift, bowel and continence care, bathing one in bed, vigilance regarding skin care to prevent pressure sores, management of a special diet and feeding the client. Formulate wages based upon credentials. A caregiver providing services at this level should have professional training, such as that of a certified nursing assistant, or a licensed practical nurse.

Injury prevention for both the senior and caregiver are always a priority. Continuing education is essential to reduce stress and prevent injury in the task of caregiving provision. The caregiver must not step beyond the limits within which his/her credentials apply. The best caregivers are those who take care of themselves. Stay physically fit, eat nutritiously and include stress reducing activities into your own lifestyle.

Caregiving for the elderly can be an enriching experience. Each client and family member will become a source of learning. This service-provision career gives back a personal opportunity to vicariously feel the spice of life as aging commences. To observe how each senior lives the precious final moments of time in his/her own individual way, will change our way of thinking about how we use time, manage our personal health and treat each other on a daily basis.

Chapter 11

Information regarding Diagnoses

CAREGIVERS NEED TO BE PROACTIVE in learning about the diagnoses seniors present. Continuing education should be a part of the caregiver's business format. The cost of continuing education is usually tax deductible. Enhanced qualifications will be useful during a crises or emergency. A caregiver who lists additional credentials on his/her résumé will gain greater marketing options.

The following articles provide information regarding some of the most common diagnoses found in the senior population. These articles will help the family and caregiver understand how a particular disease process can affect a senior's quality of life. (See the Glossary below.)

Alzheimer's Disease

A local photographer was hired to record an event at a skilled care nursing facility. The photographer was interacting with the staff and residents to organize photographic opportunities. One resident wheeled up to the photographer, pulled on his sleeve and stated "Excuse me, you look like you know everybody here, can you tell me who I am?"

Alzheimer's disease is a slow progressive disorder that results in loss of memory, language and thinking skills. The disease also affects judgment and personality, resulting in behavioral changes. The atmosphere to establish when working with clients with a cognitive impairment such as dementia or Alzheimer's disease is one that is safe and secure, calm and reassuring. The client with Alzheimer's disease is like a vulnerable child. As caregivers we must not treat them like children, but intuitively help them to feel completely safe and without fear or anxiety.

Alzheimer's disease is progressive. The stages listed below describe changes that occur as someone with this type of disease declines in health.

Level 1

Hiring a caregiver at this level will provide benefits of early intervention.

> Forgetfulness, may not be taking medications as directed
> Intermittent losses of awareness of time, day and place
> Impaired judgment with evidence of social improprieties
> Out of touch in social gatherings
> Lack of spontaneity, or the opposite: overexcited and impulsive
> Apathy (inability to feel pleasure)
> Decreased motivation for activities once enjoyed
> Shortened attention span
> Diminished ability to plan, manage finances, organize events, and do housekeeping tasks or meal prep
> Decreased capacity to perform basic activities of daily living including regular grooming and hygiene
> Growing number of incidents of incontinence (urinary and/or bowel)

Level 2

Full-time care around the clock will be required at this level.
> Restlessness, pacing, wandering
> Repeating questions or stories (perseveration)
> Feeling disoriented in places once familiar
> Social disorientation in the presence of people once close to them (even family members)
> Increased forgetfulness; loss of awareness of time
> Agitation, confusion, anxiety (may be noted more at night)
> Sensory sensations may become inhibited: sense of touch, vision, proprioception (loss of awareness of placement of feet may create difficulty in walking or shuffling)
> Inability to filter out background noise
> Inability to understand long sentences or verbal instructions be-

yond step one
> Diminishing ability to initiate and manage self-care tasks
> Able to participate in social events for only a brief period; easily becomes over-stimulated
> Exhibits frustration and anger and, on occasion combative behavior
> Personality changes
> Feelings of vulnerability, including fears about personal security and basic sense of survival
> Inappropriate sexual behavior, lack of social constraints
> Growing obsession with trash; throws items away or flushes them down the toilet
> Develops speech difficulties, unable to find words or complete sentences
> Requires assistance managing grooming and hygiene tasks, as well as preparing and eating meals
> Incontinence
> Muscle weakness and weight loss may develop; possibly seizures, muscle twitching

Level 3

Care at home may become impossible; attentive caregiving required 24/7.
> Complete dependence for all self-care tasks
> Turning in bed is required every 1.5 hours to eliminate pressure sores and skin ulcers
> Senior develops a need to put things into mouth
> Speech impairment; muteness
> Loss of control of all body functions
> At great risk for falls (if still walking) due to general muscle weakness
> At risk for urinary tract infection, skin ulcers, pneumonia, bowel impaction, dehydration
> Difficulty swallowing and suffers from aspiration (drawing food into the windpipe) due to weak muscles
> Emaciation and failure of multiple body systems

These levels outline general symptoms of decline. One with dementia or Alzheimer's disease may have overlapping indicators as the disease progresses. In example: he/she may show symptoms from level 1 and level 2 simultaneously. The decline process may be slow over the course of years or it may unfold more rapidly. Alzheimer's and dementia-related diseases are complex in that the decline affects both the brain and the body. Caregiving in the face of this global type of physical and mental loss is very difficult. The caregiver may be a spouse who is grieving the loss of the loved one as they care for a very different person.

Those with dementia are often aware that they are unable to care for their own needs. This creates feelings of vulnerability. Alzheimer's patients may not recognize someone who is living with them, even a spouse. At times they will ask who family members are and they may become paranoid about the presence or actions of caregivers or family members. This type of fear may be derived from vulnerability and is a response noted in both male and female genders. A person who feels that their basic survival needs are threatened, may strike out. A spouse who is alone in the caregiving process may be in danger if the senior with dementia becomes combative out of fear or due to irrational thinking.

The signs of potential danger to self or others in relation to the behavior of one diagnosed with Alzheimer's are rarely discussed in the primary care physician's office. *In some circumstances, the caregiver dies in the process of caring for the senior with Alzheimer's diseases* (Waarala n.d.). This is a tragic outcome for those who feel a sense of duty to the family member with dementia or Alzheimer's disease. More information needs to be broadcast to the community about this complex disease as loved ones are, at times, inadvertently abused and hurt in the role of caregiver. Support for the family and caregiver(s) is needed to relieve the stress that results in negative health issues for those so closely involved in the selfless day-to-day provision of care. Any rough or uncharacteristic behaviors observed in the senior with Alzheimer's or dementia-related disease should be discussed with a geriatric specialist as soon as possible. A consultation/evaluation with a geriatric specialist can yield useful information about how best to safely support the senior with Alzheimer's at the level of care that is needed. Professional help from geriatric doctors and eldercare lawyers will inform the decision-making process. A geriatric specialist will help to determine if it is safe for the spouse or live-in caregiver to be alone with the senior who has this sort of cognitive affliction. This type of evaluation will give concrete evidence to the family that the one diagnosed with Alzheimer's disease may require the care provided in a long-term care facility for the safety and well-being of all involved.

The role of an eldercare lawyer is to assist the family in estate and financial planning needed to secure long-term care. In most circumstances, the financial security of the spouse is also maintained in this process. Make an appointment with eldercare lawyers in the early stages of Alzheimer's (see level 1 above) to assure financial support as the disease progresses.

It is not a failure to place a senior in a long-term-care facility if it is determined to be the safest and most suitable living arrangement. It is a practical outcome for one in the later stages of this type of disease. Alzheimer's disease is not curable; it is terminal.

Helpful Interventions

Family members and caregivers will find many ways to assure one with dementia or Alzheimer's disease. The following tips are suggested.

> › Reassure the senior that he/she is safe. Use a calm tone of voice without judgment.
> › Do not talk with the senior regarding the irritation if he/she becomes upset.
> › Try to lower the possibility of agitation in the future by noting what happened just prior to a particular outburst; what triggered the feelings of insecurity?
> › Remove the senior from the upsetting atmosphere; suggest a walk to another room.
> › Introduce a new thought or activity.
> › Ask the senior to help with a task he/she can manage successfully.
> › Suggest engagement in a purposeful activity such as folding clothes or looking at a picture book.
> › Calming music may soothe and put the senior at ease.

These steps may help an agitated senior feel secure and confident. *For this type of client, a routine with consistent nutritious meals is vital to keep one comfortable and aware that the caregiver will provide what is needed in a timely manner.* This brings a sense of security and will help to eliminate anxiety.

Home Security and Safety Adaptations

All areas within the living quarters of one with Alzheimer's or dementia related disease will have to be modified for safety.

> › Secure household garbage so it is not accessible to the senior.
> › Remove all poisonous and hazardous materials; secure medications in a locked cabinet.
> › Power buttons on electrical appliances, especially the stove and oven should be covered or removed to prevent fire hazard or accidental burns.
> › Microwaves may not be safe to use because they can cause burns.

> Use electrical socket covers.
> Store knives and matches and barbecue lighters out of reach.
> Sinks in kitchen and bathroom should be fitted with an open but screened drain to prevent water from overflowing, or items being washed down.
> Securely cover the toilet to prevent important items being flushed down.
> Lock outside doors in the home at all hours to prevent the senior from roaming out into the elements.
> Install bells on doors to alert the caregivers that the client is wandering.
> Keep keys (for car and other locked items), important papers and non-replaceable items out of reach; those with dementia or Alzheimer's are prone to hiding things.
> Close off stairways or areas of the house that are not being used. Lock if necessary.
> A caregiver should be with one with Alzheimer's or dementia at all times to prevent harmful consequences due to loss of cognitive functioning.
> Be sure smoke alarms and gas detectors are in working order.
> Follow suggestions provided throughout this book in terms of caregiving especially as one reaches the later stages of this disease.

Caregivers and family members may attend regular information seminars relative to Alzheimer's disease or dementia. Local county health departments and the Alzheimer's Association offer assistance, day care opportunities and educational support to help family members and caregivers. Respite care is often necessary to decrease caregiver burnout. Ask the primary care physician or geriatric specialist about hospice care. Hospice Care is a Federal Benefit under Medicare Part A. Your loved one may qualify for these benefits. at later stages of decline.

Arthritis

Arthritis is a degenerative disease that requires careful management. There are many types of arthritis. This article will discuss two: rheumatoid arthritis and osteoarthritis.

Rheumatoid arthritis affects the fluid of the synovial joints. Osteoarthritis affects the cartilage of the joints. Both diseases can cause joint contractures and limit ROM. Hip and knee replacement surgery may be necessary for those with arthritis as weight-bearing joints break down with normal use.

Inflammation of joints indicates that arthritis has reached an *acute phase*. Signs of inflammation are red, swollen hands, knees, or ankles and expressed pain. When inflammation or pain is observed, follow an energy-conservation routine with paced increments of ADL's. Tasks should be no longer than 10 to 15 minutes at a time and no lifting or heavy activity should be done. The senior will need to focus energy on basic activities of daily living with no extra-curricular activities while experiencing the pain and low energy of the acute phase. Pushing through taxing activities will only increase the pain and exacerbate the disease process.

Precautions to take when working with someone with rheumatoid or osteoarthritis are as follows.

During Acute Phase

When inflammation and redness of joints are observed and the client expresses pain, he/she is experiencing an acute phase of arthritis.

> Alert family to begin anti-inflammatory medication if the senior has not done so.
> Incorporate frequent rest breaks in the daily routine.
> Keep the senior warm and comfortable.
> Use posture support when the senior is seated.
> Respect pain thresholds: inquire frequently about the intensity of pain.
> Active range-of-motion (AROM) will be completed within the routine ADL's only.
> To conserve energy, do not engage additional AROM exercises during acute phase of arthritis.
> Limit weight bearing: sit for small tasks such as making a sandwich.
> Limit or avoid engagement in tasks that pose resistance, such as, lifting pots/pans in kitchen, opening jars, pushing/pulling activities (heavy doors).
> Avoid *static hold* when reading a book; use a book rest.
> Decrease *static hold* by holding walker handles for no more than 10 minutes at a time; release one hand at a time to relax each in turn, or sit and release the hold on both handles.

As Acute Phase Diminishes

A decrease in swollen/red joints and a lower threshold of pain will indicate that the client is moving away from the acute phase of arthritis. Continue to maintain vigilance.

› Follow an energy-conservation routine allowing paced increments of ADL's: limit tasks to 45 minutes when arthritic joints are not inflamed, to prevent the return of an acute phase.

› AROM will be completed within the routine ADL's; additional AROM exercises may be engaged as tolerated in seated position.

› Rest breaks should be taken every 30 to 45 minutes.

› Engage senior in activities of interest and in social interactions to reduce stress.

› Follow any exercises as directed by the home healthcare providers only as tolerated when arthritic joints are not inflamed, to prevent the return of an acute phase.

› Follow suggestions for sleep hygiene in Chapter 4, "Applying the Care Plan," to insure as much restful sleep as possible each night.

› To prevent a relapse, continue with these tips even when the acute phase is not active.

Joints that are afflicted with any arthritic condition may become deformed due to a breakdown in the structure of the joint capsule (contracture). Any structural change will result in a permanent loss of joint ROM. While this condition cannot be corrected through stretches and exercise, it is important to maintain the ROM that is available through engagement of ADL's and any additional active ROM exercises prescribed by the home healthcare providers as tolerated by the senior.

Diabetes

Type 1 diabetes is a disease in which a person is insulin deficient. The pancreas is not producing insulin and the individual is unable to metabolize sugar. The results are high blood sugar (glucose) levels.

Type 2 diabetes is a disease in which a person is able to produce insulin but has lower levels of insulin or the insulin is unable to complete the task of metabolizing sugar. This also results in high blood sugar (glucose) levels.

Successful management of Type 1 or Type 2 diabetes requires timing and consistent meal intake following a guided plan per individual needs. This must be organized within the daily routine. For example, meals should be eaten at the same time approximately each day, even if traveling outside of the home.

One with diabetes will need counseling regarding how to eat and manage sugar and carbohydrate intake with the support of prescription insulin or with diet alone. A *diabetes care specialist* will recommend the preferred types of food for this diagnosis as well as organizing food intake intervals. An *endocrinologist* will provide individual guidance regarding the management of insulin. Referrals for these specialists will be provided by the primary care physician.

Blood glucose levels need to remain within a specific level as tested by a glucose monitor. Glucose readings between 70 to 140 milligrams per deciliter are considered normal.

> 70 is the lowest normal glucose level.
> 140 is the highest normal glucose level.
> It is life threatening if sugar levels drop below 70, or increase beyond the normal range of 140.
> Low sugar levels (below 60) may lead to a state of unconsciousness and seizures.

Always take a travel pack when out with a senior with diabetes. This should hold a glucose monitor, insulin, snacks and glucose tablets.

Indications of Low Blood Sugar

A person experiencing low blood sugar or hypoglycemia will demonstrate the following signs.

> Slurred speech
> Expressed low energy, crabby and irritable mood
> Pale complexion
> Slow response to questions
> Nervousness or anxiety
> Lightheadedness or dizziness
> Report of visual limitations, such as, tunnel vision or poor long-distance vision

If low blood sugar is suspected, keep the senior seated and provide quick intervention. Check blood for glucose level. If glucose level is below 70 administer a snack: fruit, banana, orange juice or glucose tablet as quickly as possible. It takes more than 35 minutes for the snack or glucose tablet to take effect. Keep the senior seated until they report feeling better, and speech is clear. For anyone in this condition who slips into a comatose condition, call 911 immediately. Do not try to administer juice, food or a glucose tablet.

High Glucose Levels

In contrast consistently high glucose levels have a long-term negative effect on the kidneys, optic nerve, and circulation. Poor circulation in one with diabetes will result in swelling in lower limbs and hands and an inability to heal sores on extremities. Complications related to poor circulation are pressure sores at bony prominences or open sores on toes or feet. Extra vigilance can prevent complications related to high glucose levels. Observe and clean the senior's feet no fewer than four times a week. Examine and note any redness or open sores. Comfortable shoes with moisture absorbent socks will help to prevent blisters. If swelling is noted in legs or feet, keep feet elevated while in a seated position.

Additional problems that result secondarily from diabetes are neuropathy, urinary tract infection, and dry skin.

Neuropathy, presents as nerve pain in the hands, legs and feet, and manifests in any range of sensations, from pain to numbness and weakness. Neuropathy makes it difficult to walk or engage in ADL's.

Urinary tract infection is common in those with diabetes, due to sugar circulating in the blood and urine. This may be further aggravated if dehydration occurs. Provide plenty of water throughout the day and encourage your client to drink frequently for rehydration purposes and to prevent infections and dry skin. Moisturize skin frequently, after bathing and/or during dressing.

Report any of the above findings immediately to the family. If an open sore is present, action must be taken. The primary care physician or geriatric specialist will need to intervene with infections or open sores. A podiatrist is an essential team member in the care of a person with diabetes and will make recommendations regarding foot care, as well as manage pedicure needs. The primary care doctor may refer a visiting nurse for wound care at home and family/caregiver training.

A successful individualized plan for diabetes control will need to be organized within the daily routine. One with diabetes cannot rely on insulin injections alone to control blood glucose levels. Exercise on a regular daily basis will improve circulation and, in some cases, improve glucose metabolism. Exercise in combination with consuming high quality foods are essential. The types of food that are recommended include non-processed whole foods, protein, complex carbohydrates, fruits and vegetables. See "Food as Fuel," in the next article for helpful tips. Incorporating these interventions into the care-plan routine will help establish a supportive health intervention for one with diabetes.

Recent research regarding insulin intolerance in the brain indicates a correlation between diabetes and dementia or Alzheimer's disease. Evidence shows that insulin intolerance or impaired ability for insulin to metabolize sugar may be found in single organ areas of the body. If the brain becomes a "target organ" of insulin intolerance the brain does not receive glucose as a required nutrient and the neuronal cells die. This creates neuron cell destruction that is similar to that found in those with advanced stages of Alzheimer's disease. Because neither Type 1 nor Type 2 diabetes is diagnosed in those with single organ insulin intolerance in the brain, the problem remains undetected during the lifetime of one with this condition. These new findings represent a brain-specific form of diabetes mellitus now being coined Type 3 diabetes (de la Monte and Wands 2008).

Food as Fuel

Weight stability is vital for our mental, physical, and emotional health. Current research indicates that some types of food we eat trigger neurotransmitters specifically identified as endorphins, serotonin and dopamine. These chemicals are natural opiates that induce pleasure or a calming effect. The release of endorphins, serotonin, and dopamine is a reaction similar to that which is generated as a result of addictive drug use (Willett 2010, 7–10). In other words, certain types of foods ingested may result in addictive cravings because they cause a chemical pleasure response, while at the same time, leave one feeling unsatisfied, hungry and reaching for more unhealthy snacks and beverages.

As children, we are encouraged to ingest food to soothe our emotions or as a reward for positive behavior. It is difficult to unravel the emotional baggage impressed upon us from environmental upbringing and modern-day, food-related influences such as TV advertising, special events, family gatherings, reward systems, strip mall fast food locations, to name a few. To clear away unhealthy developed habits and fight off the overload of information, counseling is advised if weight gain or loss is a problem. It is also helpful to establish an understanding of food as fuel. Food is not a reward, entertainment process nor is it intended to soothe our emotions. Even though it does all this and more we must begin to see food in practical terms: *the primary role of food in our lives is to fuel, energize and keep our body and brain healthy and alive. This is the food/fuel/energy process.*

The food/fuel/energy process is complex and individual nutritional needs, as well as food intake education, are best recommended by a nutritionist so that we learn how our body uses and stores food. The daily necessity of sustenance makes it impossible to go "cold turkey" and "just say no" to food if we are trying to lose weight. Planning meals as well as using self-discipline need to become a daily practice in order to maintain balanced weight.

Smart grocery shopping for healthy food is a priority. This means that our cooking has to go beyond opening and consuming boxed, processed, packaged foods. A good cookbook and learning to cook from scratch are the tools we need to create nutritional meals. All foods may be enjoyed in moderation, yet it is imperative that eating habits follow proper nutritional recommendations to balance sustenance with some pleasure foods.

As noted above, scientific research has begun to label immoderate food consumption as an addiction. Artificial chemicals (preservatives, food colorings, artificial flavors, and aromas) as well as excessive amounts of salt or sugar (natural and artificial) all contribute to the disruption of the normal state of our food/fuel/energy process. Foods that are most addictive are typically processed, may have a gratifying texture, and are high in sugar, salt and fat content. These foods are designed to be pleasing to the taste, very palatable, and thus seem to be most rewarding. Studies have found, however, that the cycle of overindulging in low-quality processed foods — no matter how palatable they may be — results in craving more food. In stark contrast, *foods that are more natural and less processed are also flavorful, yet they do not create the same cravings as processed items, because they are satiating.*

Some ways to break this cycle are to eat complex carbohydrates and lean protein. These foods have been found to promote satiation. When complex carbohydrates are eaten separately, they boost alertness and decrease stress. When complex carbohydrates are eaten in combination with lean protein, the results are sustained energy, improved mood, as well as decreased stress (Willett 2010, 27–29). Complex carbohydrates also help to keep insulin levels in balance. Complex carbohydrates help us to feel satiated and will prevent loss of control when we have gone a while without food, or are trying to limit intake of simple carbohydrates. *The dietary change is not to eat less but to eat more satiating foods in moderate proportions, while cutting back on processed foods.*

Many foods have complex carbohydrates in them. They are called nutrient-dense foods. Some examples are: foods lean or low in solid fats, (solid at room temperature, e.g., butter), fish and poultry, all vegetables and fruits, fat-free or low-fat milk and yogurt, eggs, beans and nuts, pasta made from whole grain flour.

Another type of food essential for daily nutrition is whole grains. Grains that are described as "whole" indicate that the bran and germ have not been removed through processing. Studies show that eating whole grain foods, specifically rich in essential fatty acids, B vitamins and minerals, nourishes the brain (Pawlak n.d.). To counteract feelings of hunger we need to consume one half of our daily grain serving as whole grain foods. Examples of foods from whole grains are: buckwheat, bulgur wheat, millet, oatmeal, quinoa, rolled oats, brown or wild rice, whole grain barley, whole rye, and whole wheat. Another benefit of eating these foods is that they have naturally occurring fiber in their makeup.

Other food necessities are plenty of fruits, vegetables (five to six servings a day) and moderate amounts of low-fat dairy items, plus 6 to 8

(8-ounce) glasses of water each day.

In summary, we feel satiated most if we eat wholesome grains and cereals, bread or pasta made from non-refined flour, fruits, vegetables. Add healthy protein like beans, nuts, fish, eggs, poultry and you begin to fuel the body for long-term energy. We begin to feel better physically, emotionally and mentally.

It is necessary to maintain improved eating patterns long enough to correct poor eating habits. Changing habits may take up to four or five months and will require long-term vigilance and self-discipline to control food intake during this time (O'Brien 2009, 326–55).

The above information does not cover all the daily food recommended requirements for healthy nutrition. If weight control is a problem or energy levels are low, ask your primary care physician for a referral to a nutritionist for an individualized consultation regarding nutrition. Also, see the many books available on healthy eating and nutrition.

Proper nutrition alone will not result in balanced weight. Exercise and daily activities that increase metabolism are also key to maintaining balanced weight. Simple walking increases metabolism as it enhances mood and decreases appetite. Add extra walking into your lifestyle, for example, park at a safe distance away from shopping locations and walk to shop. Use stairs instead of the elevator. Stand to do some tasks. These activities, when incorporated into a regular routine, will increase metabolism.

The more caregivers increase their knowledge about suitable foods the more they will be able to help seniors form a daily routine around proper nutrition and exercise. Good nutrition and exercise translates into physical strength, cognitive clarity, mood stability and improved sleep. Remember to get approval from your primary care physician before beginning any changes in diet or an exercise routine.

Special Senses

Vision Loss

Those with visual difficulties beyond what may be corrected by prescription glasses will need to have adaptive touch/tactile information added to the home environment and personal items. This will assist in building a "mental map" of the living space as the senior "reads" the tactile information identifying all needed household and personal items. An example is raised markers on microwave buttons to indicate various cooking options. This is as simple as placing raised tape on the most frequently used buttons. Sew tactile markers into the individual's clothing as a means of identification for outfit choices.

The home healthcare providers will assist in modifying the home for easy accessibility and the use of stove top, microwave and conventional ovens. This assessment will include the safe use of other home appliances, as well as communication devices/adaptive equipment.

The family will adapt and maintain the home environment for safe accessibility based on the home healthcare provider's recommendations. Once the living space is set for the senior with low vision or no vision, the environment must be maintained. The smallest variation in the environment will create a safety hazard. Anyone coming in and out of the home must not move anything. The senior's routine and mental mapping must be respected at all times by visitors or anyone who shares the living space.

Community resources such as audio books are available from the community library. State and county agencies provide services and resources for the blind within the area of the senior's home.

The family and caregiver will need to be vigilant to maintain safety requirements and organize the environment of one with low vision or blindness. Begin in the kitchen. Keep the number of utensils and pots and pans to a minimum. Mark all needed utensils, dishes and pots and pans with tactile identifiers. Store only what is needed in cupboards and on shelves. Organize like items with like items. This will support an easy mental map configuring the location of items. Place all needed items within easy reach. Clean out the refrigerator frequently and organize a means of marking items for the senior to identify readily.

Toiletries and bathroom necessities will need tactile marking and to be stored in specific locations. Both the bathroom and kitchen will need to be sanitized daily to maintain clean utensils, counters and utilitarian surfaces. One with low vision will not be able to see dirt particles easily.

Medications must be monitored and carefully marked for easy identification. Assistance may be necessary if the senior is not able to safely manage this task independently. A medical alert system for emergency intervention must be in place if the senior is living alone. Phones and communications devices must be adapted and within easy reach for instant use. All exits must be fully accessible at all times with no clutter throughout the living quarters to make the senior's "mental map" easy to maintain and safe.

In addition to these recommendations, it is important to remain vigilant to seasonal changes. Window air conditioners in summer and extra blankets in bedrooms in winter may become hazards. Introduce these changes to the senior for orientation and adjustment in his/her mental map. Remember to change lamps activated on a timer as the seasonal solstice and equinox lighting changes, as well as clock settings when daylight savings time requires.

Hearing Loss

Hearing loss is a difficult impairment. There is a lack of awareness of what is happening to the sides as well as behind the one afflicted. Also, the social isolation that coincides with this sensory loss is comparable to an abysmal sentence within solitary confinement. Communication is vital and paramount in the survival of all humans; yet a hearing impairment makes it difficult if not impossible to hear and thus grasp the content of ordinary conversations.

One with this affliction will need some means of acquiring "eyes" behind their back to gain awareness of what may be coming their way. While ambulating, a caregiver will need to remain close to the client to assure that such clues from behind are received and will not catch one with a hearing loss off guard.

Home Accommodations for the Hearing Impaired

The following modifications will increase communications and decrease isolation.

> Phones will need to be adapted with light and vibration to alert of an incoming call; as well as speaker boost.
> The caregiver's companionship becomes all the more important in this situation because isolation and a lack of social engagement become a quality-of-life issue for those with hearing impairment.
> A hearing aid, headphones for use with televisions and music equipment, and audio books all strengthen the senior's connection with the community and assist in safety.

Home healthcare providers will assist in modifying the home for easy accessibility and instruct the senior and family members in the use of communication devices and adaptive equipment as needed. Lights will help in announcing incoming communications via phone, or if someone is at the door.

Loss of Special Senses as a Result of Cerebral Vascular Accident

Losses of special senses can occur as a result of a stroke (cerebral vascular accident) or other brain injury. The home healthcare providers will assess the specific needs of the senior in this circumstance. The list that follows indicates possible problem areas.

Tactile sensibility is the awareness of textures and various forms or shapes of material items that we grasp in our hands and feel through touch.

The loss of this type of information will decrease the ability to know that we are holding something, or to identify what we have in our hand. Grasping, holding, and lifting are difficult when tactile sensibility is lost. Handling hot items in the kitchen would be off limits for one with this condition. Microwave may be possible with proper containers that do not conduct heat, with the use of pot holder mitts. Check the senior's skin condition frequently.

Hot and cold perception is the ability to determine the temperature of items. With this sensory loss it is difficult for one to dress suitably for specific climate temperatures and conditions. Winter clothing will be needed for outdoor traveling. Extra blankets placed on extremities will be needed at rest, or one who is routinely in a wheelchair. A moderately cool temperature should be maintained in the summer; plus lots of drinking water. The stove would be off limits for one with this condition. Microwave may be possible with proper containers that do not conduct heat, with the use of pot holder mitts. A caregiver must always be mindful of the need to maintain safe food temperatures and adjust the thermostat for a comfortable in-home climate. The bath water must be monitored for safety as well.

Proprioception is an unconscious awareness of one's position in space due to sensory feedback from muscles, tendons and joints regarding movement. This message is transmitted through a sensory mechanism called the golgi tendon organ, which reacts when the muscles stretch. As one moves out of the base of gravity, the muscles will register an exaggerated stretch. This will create a reflexive reaction to shorten the muscle and recoil to prevent injury. A lack of proprioceptive awareness in the legs/feet will create instability in walking, and balance problems with the possibility of falling. Another related problem is that one with a lack of proprioception awareness may not move to adjust position while seated in a chair or during sleep. This can lead to pressure sores, usually at bony prominences. This is a problem for anyone who must remain in a seated position, such as in a wheelchair or lying in bed, for long lengths of time. Seniors should be reminded to move frequently. If unable to move on their own, he/she will have to be repositioned every 1.5 hours.

Neuropathy is misinformation transferred by the peripheral nervous system from the extremities: legs, feet, arms, and hands. The information perceived by the client will be any range of sensation from pain and tingling to numbness. This creates a lack of coordination. Those with diabetes frequently express this nerve pain or tingling in feet or hands. When it occurs in the feet or lower legs, walking is difficult due to a lack of awareness of where feet are in support of one's weight, or loss of confidence in stability. If neuropathy occurs in the hands, it will be difficult to hold items or use tools.

The sense of smell may be diminished in the elderly. If this occurs, they may have a decrease in appetite because the aroma of food is a great part of taste. Another difficulty may be the inability to smell a gas leak, smoke or other various noxious odors that alert one to danger. This would require vigilance on the part of the family and caregiver. Add smoke detectors and gas and carbon monoxide detectors to the residence and check the battery frequently.

Vestibular or balance may be compromised due to a cerebrovascular accident or other type of brain injury. The home healthcare providers will assess and provide specific safety measures to be maintained during ambulation and ADL task process.

Glossary

Active Range-of-Motion (AROM)
The amount of movement at any joint when one performs activities without assistance. The flexibility available at joints as one moves through daily tasks. The amount of movement at a joint when moved voluntarily by the senior.

Adaptive Equipment
Tools used to provide leverage or assistance in completing tasks. Examples are: a cane to assist in walking; a reacher (stick with grip) to grasp and hold items out of reach; an adjustment in the handle of a tool resulting in supportive grip strength and improved leverage.

ADL's
Acronym describing activities of daily living. These include personal self-care, grooming/hygiene, dressing, bathing, oral hygiene, meal preparation, taking medications, communicating with friends/family, social/leisure activities, occupation/employment.

Advanced Directives
Legal documents, such as a living will or advanced directives for medical care or finances. These documents are organized in advance of a condition that renders the person unable to make medical decisions for themselves if one becomes incapacitated. Such advanced directives will identify a specific person to be the health care proxy or agent who will have legal ability to make decisions on behalf of that person. These documents describe preferences regarding end-of-life care and financial management.

Ambulate
To walk or move about from place to place independently, with a cane, walker or wheelchair.

Apathy
A form of psychological detachment or an inability to experience pleasure or excitement resulting in decreased motivation for daily activities and a lack of quality of life.

Arthritis
A disorder of the joints where the synovial fluid or the joint capsule is diminished, resulting in pain and inflammation at the joints afflicted. Arthritis occurs as a consequence of an autoimmune disease or previous injury.

Osteoarthritis
A form of arthritis in which inflammation of the joint coverings and cartilage of specific joints causes bone and cartilage degeneration.

Rheumatoid Arthritis
Inflammation of the synovial fluid in joint capsules of specific joints; this leads to the breakdown of specific joints. This is an autoimmune disease.

Fibromyalgia
A chronic disorder affecting the muscles; while not involving the joints, it is similar to arthritis in that it results in pain and fatigue and irregular sleep patterns. A chronic disorder in which the musculoskeletal system is afflicted with pain, inflammation and tenderness. Fatigue and weakness is present and causes a decrease in one's ability to manage daily tasks.

Aspiration
Drawing food particles or liquid into the wind pipe (trachea).

Autoimmune Disease
Disease arising when the immune system attacks and destroys parts of the body, body fluids or connective tissue.

Autonomic Nervous System
The involuntary part of the nervous system which is largely unconscious; it moderates and activates functions such as digestion, breathing, heartbeat, and other reflexive body activities.

Circadian Rhythm
An internal clock directing 24-hour intervals in mammals and most living creatures. It regulates active hours of the day as well as sleeping/eating patterns. This internal clock responds to variations of light/darkness and temperature.

Contracture
The shortening of a muscle or tendon around a joint decreasing the ROM and stability at the joint.

Durable Power of Attorney for Finances
A person chosen to make decisions on behalf of a senior regarding his/her financial management in the situation of an incapacitating medical condition. This is an *advanced directive* where terms are drawn up while the person is of sound mind and able to make his/her own decisions. The senior's wishes regarding his/her financial management is discussed with the chosen Durable Power of Attorney for Finances *in advance* of the senior's mental/physical decline.

Durable Power of Attorney for Health Care Decisions (Health Care Advocate Agent)
A person chosen to speak on behalf of the senior in the situation of an incapacitating medical condition. The health care agent will establish the senior's wishes in terms of life support and other health care issues *in advance* of the senior's mental/physical decline. When the attending or treating doctor determines that the senior is no longer able to make health care choices the health care advocate or agent will make decisions as previously directed by the senior.

Early Intervention
Proactive steps taken to prevent or eliminate a problem before it becomes more complex. An example, in regard to the senior, is hiring caregivers to support a safe approach to routine tasks before health declines. This may prevent a fall or other accidents.

Empathy
The ability to understand the feelings or the situation of another person.

Home Healthcare Providers
A team of professionals prescribed by the primary care physician to visit patients at home after discharge from a hospital stay. This team will evaluate the safety of the home and make recommendations to keep the patient improving and maintaining his/her health. The team usually consists of a nurse, occupational, and physical therapist, social worker and speech-language pathologist.

Kyphosis
A deformity in the spinal column at the cervical area (neck) creating an exaggerated forward curvature or hump.

Neurodegeneration
The loss of function within the neurons, including death of neurons.

Neuron
The nerve, the nerve cell and extended fiber.

Neuropathy
A condition in the peripheral nerves resulting in pain, tingling, numbness. These uncomfortable sensations interrupt normal tactile and pressure sensation. This creates problems in walking due to a loss of pressure sensation in feet/legs or in using hand tools due to a loss of tactile awareness.

Parasympathetic Nervous System
That part of the autonomic nervous system that involuntarily manages the internal organs, blood vessels and glands. It activates digestion and initiates restful recuperation of the body.

Peripheral Nervous System
There are two main parts of the nervous system, the central nervous system: the nerves that are located within the brain and spinal cord, and the periph-

eral nervous system. The peripheral nervous system is that part of the nervous system that is outside of the brain and spinal cord. The peripheral nervous system connects the central nervous system to parts of the body such as muscles.

Perseveration
A repetitive action, behavior or speech pattern in which one goes over the same motions or makes the same verbal statements in a repetitive manner.

Pressure Sore
The breakdown of skin around a bony prominence due to pressure and the loss of circulation in that area.

Proprioception Awareness
An unconscious awareness of one's position in space due to sensory feedback from muscles and joints regarding movement. This message is transmitted through a sensory mechanism called the golgi tendon organ which reacts when the muscles stretch. A lack of proprioceptive awareness in the muscles and joints of the legs/feet will create instability in walking, and balance problems.

Scoliosis
A lateral (side-to-side) curvature of the spine. This may cause rotation of the vertebral column.

Sleep Hygiene
Methods used to enhance sleep such as: exercise and drink plenty of water early in the day; keep stimulating electronics out of the bedroom; low lighting for safety only; decrease caffeinated drinks to early morning only; eat nutritious meals; balance activities with rest periods during the day.

Standby Assistance
A person who assists the senior only as needed allowing the senior to do what he/she is able to do safely. The person caring for the senior will stay close by (on the weaker side of the senior) to be ready to assist as needed.

Static Hold
The process of holding or supporting an object for long lengths of time. This is a type of isometric muscle contraction. Cumulative trauma to the arm and or hand may result if the practice of holding or supporting objects for long lengths of time is habitual.

Sundowner's Syndrome
A state of confusion and anxiety in some people with dementia or Alzheimer's disease. One experiencing this may become agitated at night or as darkness ensues. One with Sundowner's Syndrome may have sleeplessness and wandering at night.

Sympathetic Nervous System
That part of the autonomic nervous system that involuntarily activates the body for the fight or flight response. It increases heart rate and is active in maintaining the body's homeostasis.

Synovial Joints
The joints in the body that are surrounded by capsules and lubricated with synovial fluid. This is the most common type of joint in the body.

Vestibular System
A sensory mechanism located in the inner ear that detects movement of the head and controls balance through the head-righting mechanism located within the semi-circular canals.

References

Hopkins, Helen L., and Helen D. Smith. 1978. *Willard and Spackman's Occupational Therapy*. 5th ed. J.B. Lippincott, 134–40.

de la Monte, Suzanne M., and Jack R. Wands. 2008. "Alzheimer's Disease Is Type 3 Diabetes — Evidence Reviewed." *Journal of Diabetes Science and Technology* 2 (6): 1101–13

O'Brien, Mary. 2009. *Weight Perfect*: Biomed Books. 324–33.

Pawlak, Laura. 2009. *Stop Gaining Weight*. Jeblar, Inc.

Waarala, Carol. 2013. "A Caregiver's Travel Guide: The Alzheimer's Journey." Seminar presentation, Gentiva Hospice, Southfield, Mich.

Willett, Gina. 2010. *Food Addictions, Overeating and Mood Swings*. Institute for Natural Resources..

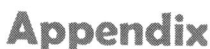

Appendix

Family/Caregiver Work Sheets

Caregivers may reproduce the six work sheets below for their personal use in caregiving. Please leave the copyright notice intact.

1. Senior's Health Journal
2. Caregiver's Daily Documentation
3. Care Plan
4. Medication List
5. Hospitality Notes
6. Contact Information

Senior's Health Journal

Morning: wake up time_____. Sleep was comfortable for____hours.

Restless for____hours.

Sugar level_____. Insulin dose _____

Medications _____

Breakfast _____

Ate breakfast at____o'clock.

List and describe any pain _____

Medication taken to relieve pain _____

Morning wash-up _____

Brush teeth _____

Dress _____

_____

Midday: Sugar level_____. Insulin dose _____

Medications _____

Lunch_____

Ate lunch at____ o'clock.

Activity/Outings _____

_____

_____

Other events _____

_____

_____

_____

Evening: Sugar level_____. Insulin dose _____

Medications _____

Dinner _____

Ate dinner at____o'clock

Quiet activity before bed_____

_____

Bedtime wash-up _____

Brush teeth _____

Change into pajamas _____

Nighttime medications _____

Snack before bed_____ ate snack at (time) _____

Bedtime _____

Reminders

» Use correct posture and abdominal muscles for rising from chair, walking or sitting.

» Take plenty of breaks.

» Drink plenty of water through the early part of day.

» Take part in daily activities that are *safe* for you as much as possible.

» Exercise following home health care providers instructions.

» Enjoy social events and activities of interest.

» Ask for help to organize your living space to prevent loss of items or falls.

» Return items to storage areas.

» Maintain healthy routine.

Caregiver's Daily Documentation

Caregiver arrival time_____ o'clock.

Climate/condition of house_____

Senior's physical condition_____

_____

_____

Senior's mental/emotional condition _____

_____

_____

Routine activities completed by the senior (ADL's) _____

_____

_____

Medications taken and at what time _____

_____

_____

How medication is prepared for the senior and by whom _____

_____

_____

Meals provided or prepared by senior _____

What the senior actually ate _____

Duties the caregiver completes _____

_____

_____

_____

Other services provided _____

_____

_____

_____

Any problems the senior demonstrated or expressed_____

_____

Instructions provided by contact person or family member related to

senior health or household issue _____

_____

_____

Action taken in response to the problem _____

_____

_____

What the senior was doing as caregiver leaves _____

_____

_____

Precautions taken before leaving the senior (accident prevention)__

_____

_____

_____

Caregiver departure time____ o'clock.

Care Plan

Senior's name _____

Phone number _____

Address _____

_____

Primary contact person _____

Phone number _____

Address _____

_____

Secondary contact person _____

Phone number _____

Address _____

_____

Permission is granted to leave messages regarding the senior on voice mail: ___yes [or] ___no

Communications Tools Checklist

» Set up calendar centrally located for senior and team to access

» Identify documentation tools and a storage place for confidentiality

» List contact person(s) numbers by the phone, plus trusted household repair person

» Contact person formulates a group e-mail system for quick dispatch of information

» Set up a phone system that the senior is able to use

» Set up emergency alert system for the senior who lives alone

Family Responsibilities

_____

_____

_____

_____

_____

Person responsible for managing the medication and refills _____

_____

_____

Level of functioning as described by the primary care doctor and Skill Lever Indicator _____

_____

_____

_____

ADL's the senior will perform (update as needed)_____

_____

_____

_____

Specific instructions provided by the doctor and home healthcare providers _____

_____

_____

_____

_____

Specific precautions regarding the senior's diagnoses—limitations —sensory losses _____

_____

_____

_____

Specific instructions regarding emergency intervention, include instructions regarding Do Not Resuscitate (DNR) orders if it pertains

_____

_____

_____

List specific instructions if hospice is part of the team _____

_____

_____

Caregiver Responsibilities

_____

_____

_____

_____

_____

Caregiver schedule _____

Medication List

List of all medications, eye drops and
vitamin supplements (indicate time taken).

Name of medication	Dosage amount	Time taken
1.		
2.		
3.		
4.		
5.		
6.		
7.		
8.		
9.		
10.		

List vitamins and over-the-counter medication: _____

_____

_____

List herbal remedies: _____

_____

_____

List food and medication allergies: _____

_____

_____

Hospitality Notes

How and when trash/recycle is managed and picked up_____

_____

List of specific grocery items (specialty items the senior likes and uses) _____

_____

_____

_____

List of any food allergies_____

_____

_____

Meal preparation specialties _____

_____

_____

List of specific cleaning/laundry supplies (specialty items the senior likes and uses) _____

_____

_____

Other specific household cleaning instructions _____

_____

_____

Skin care/cosmetic products, oral care items, shaving supplies, uses and procedures _____

_____

Contact Information

(Place by the phone; provide copy for caregiver.)

Primary contact _____

    Phone _____

Secondary contact _____

    Phone _____

Alternate emergency contact _____

    Phone _____

Trusted household repair person (for emergency house repairs)

_____

_____

    Phone _____

Name(s) and contact information for the senior's doctor(s)_____

_____

_____

_____

_____

Names and numbers of the senior's health care policies _____

_____

_____

_____

41465174R00061

Made in the USA
Middletown, DE
19 March 2017